Real Food
Real Results

Gluten-Free, Low-Oxalate, Nutrient-Rich Recipes

Melinda Keen

ISBN: 1517478537
ISBN-13: 978-1517478537

Printed in the United States of America

Photography: Melinda Keen
Editor: Jessica Matthews

Disclaimer: The recipes and views presented here are not intended as diagnosis, treatment, prescription or cure for any disease, mental or physical, and are not intended as a substitute for regular medical care. For diagnosis or treatment of any medical problem, consult your own physician. Always consult with your personal physician before beginning any new program or making any changes on your own. Any statements or claims about the health benefits conferred by any foods have not been evaluated by the FDA and are therefore not intended to diagnose, treat, cure or prevent any disease. The publisher and author are not responsible for any specific health needs and are not liable for any damages or negative consequences from any treatment, action, application or preparation, to any person reading or following the information in this book. The content of this book is the sole opinion of the author who is not in the medical profession therefore is not engaged to render any type of medical professional advice. The recipes and Cook's Notes reflect specifically on what has worked for the author.

ACKNOWLEDGEMENTS

First, I'd like to thank my Lord for giving me the strength and ability to overcome adversity. My path to health was revealed, and the results inspired a desire to help others who struggle with health related issues caused by food intolerances and a toxic diet.

I would also like to thank my editor, Jessica Matthews, for her valuable time and her keen eye for detail. I'm always impressed by her ability to edit so well, so quickly.

Finally, I'm forever grateful for my husband, Jeff Keen, who encouraged me when I needed it and helped in so many ways. Thank you for all those last minute grocery store trips during the testing of my recipes and for never complaining when dinner was multiple choice.

CONTENTS

INTRODUCTION

For the person reeling under a doctor's directions to avoid gluten or to avoid high oxalate foods, the task of creating family friendly nourishing meals can be overwhelming.

Gluten-containing foods are also high in oxalates. Gluten is a protein composite found in wheat and related grains including barley and rye. It causes inflammation in the small intestines of people with celiac disease. Oxalate is a chemical found in plant foods. High oxalate foods are known for causing kidney stones but they can cause many other problems in the body. Eating gluten-free and low-oxalate may sound restrictive but the recipes in this cookbook prove it doesn't have to be boring or complicated. The delicious healthy recipes in this cookbook are gluten-free and low-oxalate (40 to 50 mg each day) for those seeking to restore their health through diet.

Small changes in diet make a huge impact on health. Nutrition with real food is eating organic real foods and removing processed and refined foods as well as foods responsible for allergies and autoimmune disease. This holistic approach gives the body a chance to detoxify and reset health. It's eating for energy, to feel great, and to heal or prevent disease. Most of these meals are high in key vitamins and minerals, high in protein fiber, and do not contain the typical gluten-free products on the market.

All recipes include nutrient-dense, additive-free, wholesome foods such as fresh vegetables, grass-fed beef, wild-caught fish, and pasture-raised poultry and eggs. The three healthy fats used in these recipes are unrefined coconut oil, extra virgin olive oil, and butter made from grass-fed cows. These are the healthy fats readily available at a reasonable price. Emerging evidence suggests most people need about 50-70 percent of their diet (calories) as healthy fats. Many vital bodily functions depend on the presence of healthy fats in your diet.

Enjoy healthy original recipes that include casseroles, pastas, soups, stir-fries, and slow cooker meals. There are breakfasts, breads and crackers, main dishes, side dishes, and desserts. Being healthy does not mean you have to skip dessert!

EATING REAL

I believe that choosing foods that are as close to their natural state as possible is the key to a long healthy life. Another key part of a healthy diet is the absence of toxic chemicals. We should be eating foods that will nourish the body like clean, real, pesticide and hormone free products. This means cutting out processed foods and replacing them with natural whole foods such as dairy, fruits, vegetables, herbs, meats, and eggs. Good fats are also beneficial and should constitute half or more of the calories in a healthy diet.

Dairy

Regardless of whether you opt for raw, organic lightly pasteurized, or organic pasteurized, the full-fat version is the healthier choice. When the fat is removed from milk, what remains are a significant number of fat-soluble vitamins that can't be absorbed as well as an overabundance of lactose. I use full fat organic dairy products in my recipes, because the calcium from dairy binds with oxalates from foods so the body doesn't absorb the oxalate. Dairy contains negligible amounts of oxalate.

Fats

Most of my recipes are made with grass-fed cow's milk butter, ghee, organic unrefined coconut oil, and extra-virgin olive oil. Butter, especially from grass-fed cows, is a natural healthy alternative to unnatural and harmful hydrogenated vegetable oils, margarines and shortenings, or genetically modified oils. Coconut oil is the healthiest fat for frying and sautéing, because it can withstand high heat without chemically altering. Unrefined coconut oil has the flavor of fresh coconuts since it is not deodorized or chemically processed. It is rich in proteins, vitamins, and antioxidants. Extra-virgin olive oil is a healthy fat to include in your diet if it's not overheated. It should never be used as a frying oil. If the oil is truly extra-virgin it has a distinctive taste and is high in antioxidants. Butter, ghee, coconut oil, and olive oil contain negligible amounts of oxalate.

Fruits and Vegetables

It is best to eat fruits and vegetables grown organically, but if budget or availability restricts your choice, remove outer leaves or peels and wash thoroughly. Organic growers are prohibited from using synthetic pesticides that have harmful effects on your health. Buy fresh and ripe fruits and vegetables when they are in season. Otherwise choose frozen. Frozen produce is processed at peak ripeness and is the most nutrient-packed aside from fresh. My recipes rarely include canned vegetables. My main concern is their sodium content, as sodium is often added to help maintain the flavor of vegetables during the canning process. When I do use them, and it's usually because I can't find them fresh or frozen, I rinse them well in a colander. At times, I do choose food in jars, such as jams, simply to save time. Buying an organic product is important for health and nutrition, but just as important for low-oxalate dieters is checking the ingredients list for any high oxalate food. Fruits and vegetables have a wide range of oxalate contents. The recipes in this cookbook do not contain fruits and vegetables in the high oxalate range.

Herbs & Spices

Beyond adding flavor, herbs and spices carry unique antioxidants, phytosterols, and many other nutrient substances that help our body fight germs and boosts the immune system. Fresh herbs are more readily available during summer months, especially if you grow your own, but some do better when they are dried. Basically, fresh herbs and spices are added near the end of a dish, and dried ones are best added during the cooking so the flavor has time to infuse the whole dish. It is best to choose organic herbs and spices due to the fact that these are plants that are conventionally grown with the use of pesticides. Herbs and spices have a wide range of oxalate contents. The recipes in this cookbook do not contain herbs and spices in the high oxalate range.

Pepper comes from the fruit of the pepper plant. The peppercorns are processed two different ways. Black peppercorns are sun-dried to turn the pepper black. To produce white pepper, the outer layer is removed leaving only the inner seed. The high oxalate content of black pepper comes from the outer layer of the peppercorn. Therefore, white pepper is low in oxalate content and preferred in all of my recipes. If you prefer, small amounts of black pepper can be used in these recipes.

Salt

Sea salt and table salt have the same basic nutritional value. I use sea salt or pink Himalayan salt in my recipes because table salt is more heavily processed to eliminate minerals and usually contains an additive to prevent clumping.

Meat, Fish, and Eggs

For optimal health I choose grass-fed organic beef and lamb, pasture-raised turkey and chicken, wild-caught fish, and pasture-raised organic eggs. In order to be certified to the US Department of Agriculture's (USDA) organic standards, farms and ranches must follow a strict set of guidelines. The animals' organic feed cannot contain animal by-products, antibiotics or genetically engineered grains, and cannot be grown using pesticides or chemical fertilizers. No antibiotics or added growth hormones are allowed, and they must have outdoor access. If you prefer to replace some of the meats with pork I highly recommend you find a naturally raised, pastured source. Pork can have a lot of contaminants, including the controversial drug ractopamine, which is banned in many parts of the world. Farm-raised fish commonly contains high levels of contaminants as well. Farmed fish are fed an unnatural diet of grains and legumes. The healthiest choice is wild-caught fish. These fish tend to be higher in Omega 3 fatty acids, contain very low levels of disease, and are free from antibiotics and pesticides. All meats, fish, and eggs contain negligible amounts of oxalate.

Grains

Most of my recipes do not include grains as most grains are high in oxalates. White rice is a gluten-free grain that is low in oxalates, so I add rice to my meals on occasion. Plain cornmeal is also a gluten-free grain and sometimes listed as having low or sometimes medium oxalate content; therefore, I limit cornmeal to rare occasions or when I'm sure there are no other oxalate containing foods in my diet that day. Choosing organic guarantees these grains are not genetically modified. Genetically modified grains are engineered to withstand high amounts of herbicide and produce their own internal insecticide. With health on the line, it's best to err on the side of caution and stick with organic. The recipes in this cookbook do not contain glutinous grains in the high oxalate range. Some brands of baking powder use wheat starch to absorb moisture. It's important to choose a brand of baking powder that does not use wheat starch. Rumford and Clabber Girl brands are wheat free and aluminum free as well.

Legumes, Nuts and Seeds

Most legumes, nuts, and many seeds, are extremely high in oxalates. Lentils, coconut, and pumpkin seeds contain negligible amounts of oxalate and can be found in many of my recipes.

BREADS AND CRACKERS

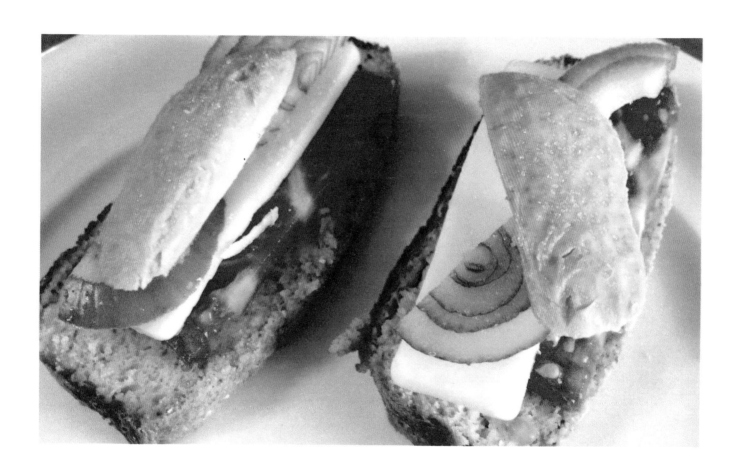

CHEDDAR CRISPS
Crunchy cheese thins packed with flavor.

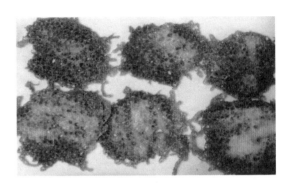

Makes 10-12
INGREDIENTS
1 cup sharp cheddar cheese, shredded
⅛ tsp. salt
⅛ tsp. white pepper
¼ tsp. onion powder
¼ tsp. garlic powder

1. Preheat oven to 425 degrees and line a large baking sheet with parchment paper. (Oil the baking sheet first so that the parchment paper lies flat.)
2. Drop large spoonfuls of cheese onto the sheet leaving about an inch of space between them. Flatten them out.
3. Mix the seasoning in a small bowl and sprinkle over each of the mounds.
4. Bake for about 7 minutes until they melt completely but have not changed color.
5. Allow to cool before transferring to a serving dish.

COOK'S NOTE
Going gluten-free doesn't have to mean cracker-free. These simple cheese crisps make a light crunchy snack or a great garnish for any dish.

NUTRITIONAL INFORMATION
Calories 44 Carbohydrate 0 g Fat 4 g Protein 3 g

COCONUT PUMPKIN BREAD

Pumpkin and coconut combine quite nicely in this sweet bread with a nutty crunch.
Serves 8

INGREDIENTS

½ cup coconut flour
1 ½ tsp. baking powder
¼ tsp. salt
6 eggs
½ cup pumpkin, cooked and mashed
½ cup maple syrup
4 tbsp. butter or coconut oil, melted
½ tsp. nutmeg
½ cup unsweetened coconut, shredded
¼ cup raw pumpkin seeds

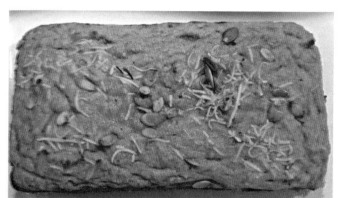

1. Preheat the oven to 425 degrees.
2. In medium-size bowl, add the coconut flour, baking powder, and salt. Mix well and set aside.
3. In a separate mixing bowl, beat the eggs; then blend in the mashed pumpkin, maple syrup, butter or coconut oil, and nutmeg. Mix well.
4. Pour wet ingredients into the dry ingredients and beat until smooth.
5. Stir in half of the shredded coconut and all of the pumpkin seeds.
6. Pour the mix into a well oiled 6x9 loaf pan and sprinkle the remaining coconut on top.
7. Bake for 35-40 minutes.
8. Allow to cool before slicing and serving.

COOK'S NOTE

Pumpkin is a fabulous source of fiber, potassium, and iron.

NUTRITIONAL INFORMATION
Calories 375 Carbohydrate 26 g Fat 29 g Protein 8 g

CORNMEAL LOAF BREAD

A healthy and delicious loaf of bread for the gluten-free sandwich lover.

Serves 8

INGREDIENTS

3 eggs, beaten
1 tbsp. maple syrup
2 cups whole milk
2 cups cornmeal, plain
1 ½ tsp. salt
1 tsp. baking soda
2 tbsp. butter, melted

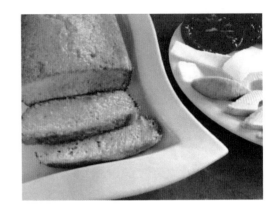

1. Preheat oven to 400 degrees.
2. In a small bowl; beat the eggs and add the maple syrup and milk. Mix well.
3. In a separate bowl, combine the cornmeal, salt, and baking soda.
4. Add the wet ingredients to the dry and pour in the melted butter. Mix until smooth.
5. Oil a 6x9 loaf pan and pour in ingredients.
6. Bake for 40 minutes and allow to cool before slicing.

COOK'S NOTE

Unlike ordinary cornbread this loaf slices well making it perfect for a healthy whole grain sandwich bread.

NUTRITIONAL INFORMATION
Calories 238 Carbohydrate 37 g Fat 7 g Protein 7 g

PIZZA CRISPS

Crunchy Italian spiced parmesan cheese thins topped with tomato and olive.

Serves 4

INGREDIENTS

1 cup parmesan cheese, shredded
⅛ tsp. salt
⅛ tsp. white pepper
⅛ tsp. onion powder
⅛ tsp. garlic powder
½ tsp. dried Italian seasonings
1 tomato, sliced thin
Black olives, sliced (as desired)

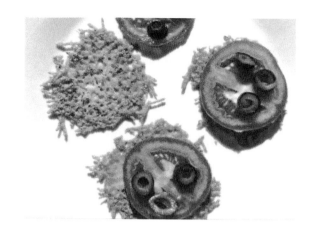

1. Preheat oven to 400 degrees.
2. Line a large baking sheet with parchment paper. You can oil the baking sheet first so that the parchment paper will lie flat.
3. Drop large spoonfuls of cheese onto the sheet leaving about an inch of space between each. Flatten them out. (Makes 10-12)
4. Add the seasonings to a small bowl, mix well, and sprinkle over the cheese.
5. Bake in a hot oven for about 6-7 minutes or until they melt completely.
6. Allow to cool before transferring to a serving dish.
7. Top with a thin slice of tomato and olive slices just before serving.

COOK'S NOTE

These flavorful crispy thins make a great snack by themselves, but the addition of tomato and olives transforms them into a tasty pizza-style appetizer.

NUTRITIONAL INFORMATION
Calories 248   Carbohydrate 4 g   Fat 16 g   Protein 22 g

SKILLET CORNMEAL CAKES

A simple southern flat cornbread with crispy edges and a delicious corn taste.

Serves 6

INGREDIENTS

2 cups yellow cornmeal, plain
2 tsp. baking powder
1 egg, beaten
1 cup water
¼ cup coconut oil (for frying)

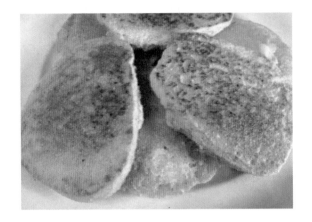

1. In a medium-size mixing bowl, combine the cornmeal, baking powder, egg, and water. Mix well.
2. In a large nonstick skillet, melt a small amount of the oil over medium-high heat and drop large spoonfuls into the oil creating about 3 cakes at a time. (Shake the skillet a bit to spread the mixture out.)
3. Cook 2-3 minutes on each side to a golden brown and remove to a plate.
4. Repeat the process to cook the remaining mix.

COOK'S NOTE

This quick flat "cornbread" is a classic deep south dish that is a delicious alternative to making a whole pan of cornbread in the oven.

NUTRITIONAL INFORMATION
Calories 286 Carbohydrate 42 g Fat 11 g Protein 5 g

SOFT DINNER ROLLS

A soft and savory grain free faux bread roll with a light texture and taste.

Serves 6
INGREDIENTS
3 eggs, separated
⅛ tsp. cream of tartar
½ tsp. honey
⅛ tsp. salt
3 oz. cream cheese

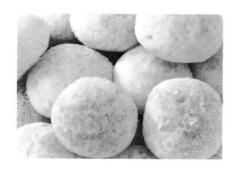

1. Heat oven to 300 degrees.
2. In a medium-size bowl, add the egg whites and cream of tartar.
3. Using an electric mixer on high, whip the egg whites until very stiff and set aside.
4. In another medium-size bowl, add the egg yolks, honey, salt, and cream cheese.
5. Using an electric mixer on high, blend until smooth.
6. Fold the egg white mixture into the yolk mixture with a spatula.
7. Spoon 6 mounds onto an oiled baking sheet.
8. Bake 25-30 minutes.
9. Cool before removing to a serving dish.

COOK'S NOTE

This light, grain free roll is so versatile. Serve it alongside any meal, or top it with anything from avocado to your favorite jam.

NUTRITIONAL INFORMATION
Calories 83 Carbohydrate 2 g Fat 7 g Protein 4 g

TAPIOCA BUNS

This soft Brazilian cheese bread is made with naturally gluten-free tapioca flour.

SERVES 6
INGREDIENTS
¼ cup coconut oil, melted
1 ½ cups tapioca flour
1 tsp. baking powder
¼ tsp. salt
2 cups cheddar cheese, shredded
2 lg. eggs

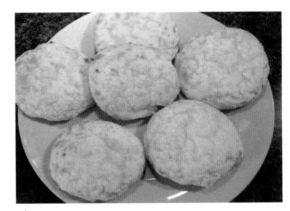

1. Preheat oven to 400 degrees.
2. Melt the coconut oil and set aside to cool.
3. In a large mixing bowl, combine the tapioca flour, baking powder, and salt.
4. Add the shredded cheese and mix well.
5. Add the eggs and the coconut oil. Mix it well with a fork at first and then by kneading. (The dough may seem too dry, but you don't want it sticky. Knead it very well. If it continues to fall apart add 1 tbsp. of water.)
6. Separate the dough into 6 equal sizes then shape each into rounds about an inch thick.
7. Place them about an inch apart on a lightly oiled baking sheet and bake at 400 degrees for 11-12 minutes. (They will flatten out some and turn a very light brown. If they get too brown they will be tough.)
8. Cool about 5 minutes before serving.

COOK'S NOTE
Tapioca buns are a wonderful, healthy replacement for hamburger buns, which are hard to find without high fructose corn syrup.

NUTRITIONAL INFORMATION
Calories 305 Carbohydrate 24 g Fat 19 g Protein 10 g

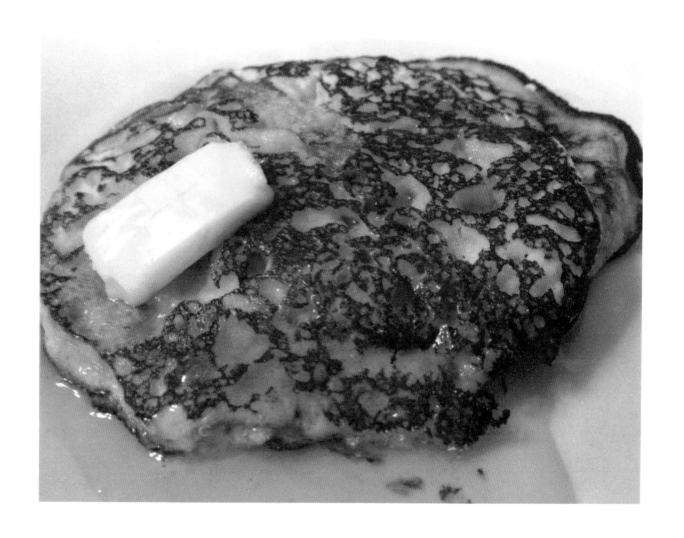

AVOCADO AND CREAM CHEESE OMELET

The warm, creamy combination of avocado and cream cheese enhances the flavor of the egg in this luscious omelet.

Serves 2

INGREDIENTS

2 eggs
1 tbsp. whole milk
¼ tsp. salt
2 tbsp. butter, 1 tbsp. per omelet
½ medium avocado, chopped
1 oz. cream cheese, chopped
Paprika (as desired)

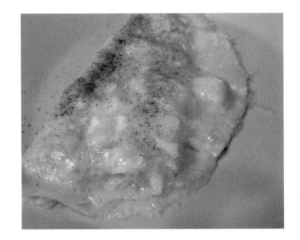

1. In a mixing bowl, whisk together the egg, milk, and salt.
2. Melt 1 tbsp. butter in a 10 or 12 inch skillet over medium heat.
3. Pour half of the egg mixture in the skillet and spread it out evenly around the bottom by rotating the skillet. Cook until done.
4. Sprinkle half of the avocado and half of the cream cheese over one half of the egg.
5. Fold the other half of the egg over the top of the avocado and cream cheese.
6. Allow the cheese a few seconds to melt; then transfer to a plate.
7. Repeat the process for the second omelet.
8. Sprinkle with paprika and serve.

COOK'S NOTE

The healthy, beneficial fats make this a blood sugar balancing breakfast.

NUTRITIONAL INFORMATION

Calories 296 Carbohydrate 6 g Fat 28 g Protein 8 g

BUTTERY BANANA MUFFINS

A moist and wholesome muffin with all natural ingredients.

Serves 6

INGREDIENTS

½ cup coconut flour
½ tsp. baking powder
1 tsp. baking soda
½ tsp. salt
5 eggs
1 cup banana, mashed
½ tsp. vanilla
2 tbsp. honey
¼ cup butter, melted

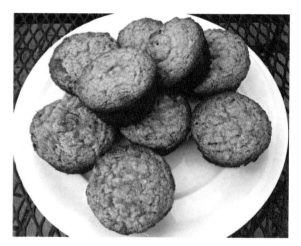

1. Preheat oven to 400 degrees and oil a 12 cup muffin pan or line with paper cupcake liners.
2. In a large bowl, mix the coconut flour, baking powder, baking soda, and salt.
3. In a separate bowl, combine the eggs, mashed banana, vanilla, honey, and melted butter. Whisk well.
4. Pour the egg mix over the coconut flour and mix well.
5. Fill muffin cups two-thirds to three-quarters full.
6. Bake for 14-15 minutes. Remove when they start to brown and a toothpick inserted in the center comes out clean.
7. Allow to cool about 5 minutes before transferring to serving dish.
8. Serve warm with a pat of butter on top.

COOK'S NOTE

Choose very ripe bananas if you desire a more intense banana flavor.

NUTRITIONAL INFORMATION

Calories 298 Carbohydrate 19 g Fat 23 g Protein 6 g

CHEESY POLENTA AND EGGS

Cheese, egg, and boiled stone-ground cornmeal create a creamy comfort food that is simple yet sumptuous.

SERVES 2

INGREDIENTS

3 tbsp. butter
½ tsp. onion powder
1 cup whole milk
½ cup stone-ground cornmeal
¼ cup cheddar cheese, shredded
2 eggs
Salt and Pepper (as desired)

1. In a large skillet, melt the butter over medium-high heat and season with onion powder.
2. In a medium-size bowl, blend the milk and cornmeal together.
3. Slowly pour the cornmeal mix into the skillet and bring it to a boil, stirring constantly.
4. Reduce heat to low and continue to simmer until it thickens, about 8-10 minutes.
5. Stir in the cheese and then open the eggs on top of the polenta keeping the yolks intact.
6. Cover and allow the polenta and eggs to cook for 4 minutes without disturbing.
7. Remove from heat and let the eggs continue to cook another minute.
8. Season with salt and pepper as desired and serve.

COOK'S NOTE
Polenta can be compared to grits, which are a southern breakfast dish in the US. Both are made from medium-grind cornmeal. It's often difficult to find organic grits, but organic stone-ground cornmeal is readily available. Stone-ground cornmeal still has the hull and the oil-rich germ of the kernel attached. It has more vitamins, minerals, and fiber. This recipe can easily be doubled.

NUTRITIONAL INFORMATION
Calories 546 Carbohydrate 39 g Fat 35 g Protein 19 g

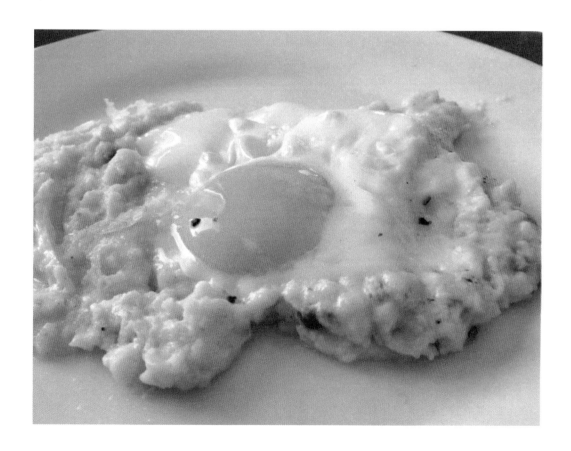

SALAD OMELET

A light and refreshing vegetarian omelet with a garden fresh salad between the folds.

Serves 2
INGREDIENTS
3 eggs
1 tbsp. whole milk
1 tbsp. onion, minced
1 tbsp. red or yellow bell pepper, minced
¼ cup cheddar cheese, shredded
1 tbsp. butter
½ cup lettuce, shredded
½ cup tomatoes, diced
Salt and pepper (as desired)

1. In a large mixing bowl, whisk the eggs.
2. Add in milk, onion, pepper, and the cheese. Mix well.
3. In a large nonstick skillet, heat the butter over medium-high heat.
4. Pour the egg mix in the skillet and rotate the skillet to spread the mixture out evenly.
5. Lower the heat to medium and cook without stirring until almost done; then remove from heat.
6. As the egg firms and cools prepare the lettuce and tomato.
7. Slide the egg to a plate and add the lettuce and tomato to one half of the egg; then fold the other half over the top.
8. Salt and pepper as desired; slice in half and serve.

COOK'S NOTE
This recipe makes a delicious light lunch or dinner as well. Each serving provides 22% of your daily requirements for vitamin K and 19% of your daily requirement for vitamin B12.

NUTRITIONAL INFORMATION
Calories 273 Carbohydrate 4 g Fat 22 g Protein 16 g

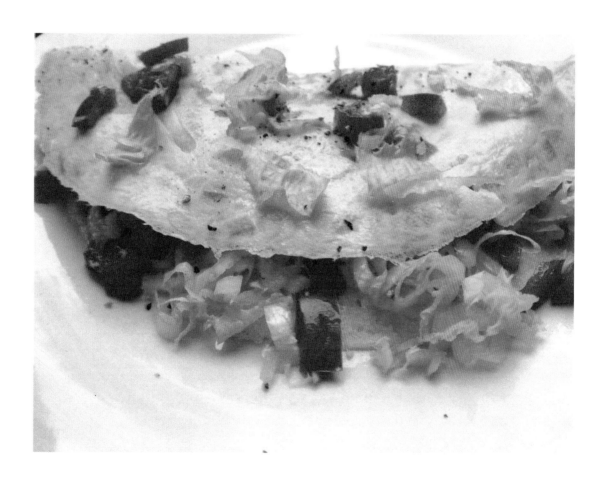

SALMON SCRAMBLE
A classic combination of creamy scrambled eggs and chunks of buttery salmon.

Serves 4-6

INGREDIENTS

5 eggs
1 tbsp. milk or cream
¼ tsp. salt
⅛ tsp. white pepper
1 tbsp. fresh chopped chives
2 tbsp. butter
14 oz. wild Alaskan salmon, drained
¼ tsp. dried dill

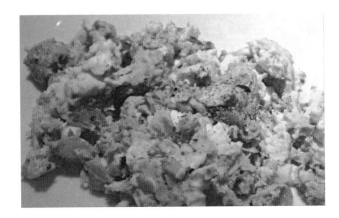

1. In a medium-size mixing bowl, combine the egg, milk, salt, pepper, and chives. Blend well.
2. In a large nonstick skillet, heat the butter over medium heat, and pour in the egg mixture.
3. Stir eggs until almost set then gently stir in and break up salmon and add the dill.
4. Continue to cook until salmon is warmed and the eggs are set.
5. Serve hot.

COOK'S NOTE

This quick and easy low-carbohydrate, protein and omega-3 rich breakfast will satisfy the heartiest appetite. Each serving supplies 64% of your daily requirement for vitamin B12 and 44% of your daily requirement for vitamin B6.

NUTRITIONAL INFORMATION
Calories 270 Carbohydrate 1 g Fat 17 g Protein 27 g

SAUSAGE

A simple recipe for making your own classic, tasty sausage patties.

SERVES 6
INGREDIENTS
1 lb. ground turkey, grass fed-beef, bison or venison

1 tbsp. white wine vinegar
1 tsp. onion powder
½ tsp. mustard seed
½ tsp. sage
½ tsp. rosemary
¼ tsp. salt
½ tsp. cayenne pepper
½ tsp. white pepper
½ tsp. garlic powder
¼ tsp. cumin
¼ tsp. chili powder
¼ tsp. fennel
2 tbsp. coconut oil (for frying)

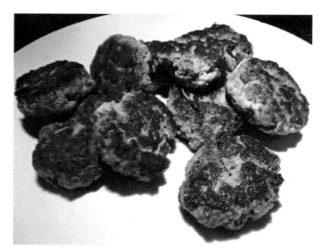

1. In a large mixing bowl, combine all of the ingredients and mix well.
2. Form patties and cook in an oiled nonstick skillet over medium-high heat until golden brown on both sides. (Makes 12 patties.)
3. Serve hot.

COOK'S NOTE
Say goodbye to all those food additives and make your own sausage. You'll never go back to buying ready-made again.

NUTRITIONAL INFORMATION
Calories 160 Carbohydrate 1 g Fat 11 g Protein 14 g

YOGURT PANCAKES

Easy, delicious, grain free and protein rich pancakes.

Serves 2
INGREDIENTS
½ cup coconut flour
¼ tsp. baking soda
¼ tsp salt
4 eggs, beaten
1 tbsp. butter, melted
1 tbsp. honey
½ tsp. vanilla
½ cup plain whole milk yogurt
3 tbsp. water
Coconut oil (for frying)
Maple syrup (as desired)

1. In a medium-size bowl, mix the coconut flour, baking soda, and salt together.
2. In a separate bowl, beat the eggs; then add the butter, honey, vanilla, yogurt, and water.
3. Pour the egg mixture over the coconut flour and mix well. Allow the mix to sit a minute or two to thicken.
4. In a large nonstick skillet, heat a small amount of coconut oil over medium heat.
5. Pour palm size cakes and shake the skillet a bit to spread them out without touching each other. (In a large skillet you can cook 2 or 3 at a time.)
6. Cook about 2-3 minutes, until bubbly on top, and then turn. Cook an additional 2 minutes or until golden brown.
7. Serve hot with maple syrup.

COOK'S NOTE
These fluffy and filling pancakes need to be cooked slowly over medium heat. The recipe can easily be doubled or tripled.

NUTRITIONAL INFORMATION
Calories 614 Carbohydrate 25 g Fat 53 g Protein 17 g

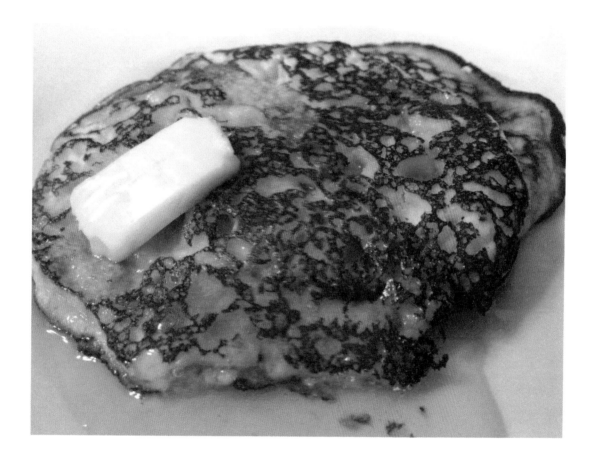

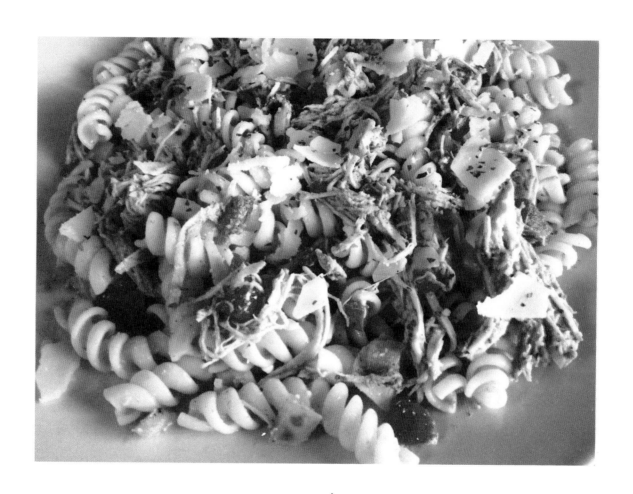

BEEF AND BUTTERNUT SKILLET
A warm and hearty meal that's also a feast for the eyes.

Serves 4
INGREDIENTS
2 tsp. coconut oil
1 medium onion, chopped
½ large red or yellow pepper, chopped
1 lb. ground grass-fed beef (or turkey, venison, bison)
3 garlic cloves, chopped
½ tsp. cayenne pepper
½ tsp. salt
½ tsp. white pepper
½ large butternut squash, cooked
1 cup cheddar cheese, grated

1. In a large nonstick skillet, heat the coconut oil over high heat. When hot, add the onion and bell pepper. Cook for about 3 minutes until soft.
2. Add the beef, garlic, cayenne, salt, and pepper, and stir-fry until the meat is browned.
3. Turn the heat down to medium and add spoonfuls of the cooked butternut squash to the skillet.
4. Stir-fry about a minute to mix the ingredients.
5. Turn off the heat and sprinkle the cheese on top.
6. Allow the cheese to melt and serve.

COOK'S NOTE

To have the butternut squash ready for this recipe, place the whole butternut squash in a slow cooker and cook on low for 6 hours or on high for 4 hours. The leftover half of the squash can be used to make a warm creamy dessert by simply adding a pinch of sea salt, some honey and butter. This delicious skillet dinner is high in vitamin C, B6, B12, niacin, and zinc.

NUTRITIONAL INFORMATION
Calories 428 Carbohydrate 16 g Fat 28 g Protein 32 g

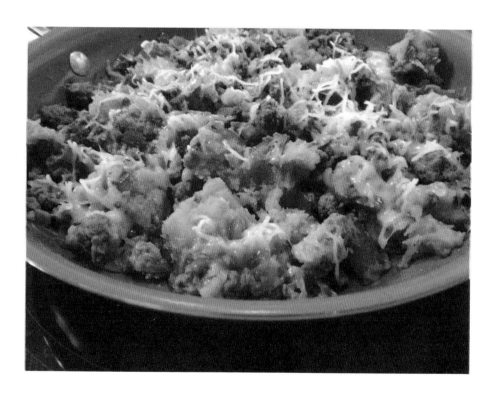

CARIBBEAN COD

A little tweak on the very traditional Jamaican dish called "Ackee and Saltfish".

Serves 4
INGREDIENTS

3 tbsp. butter
1 small onion, diced
½ red bell pepper, diced
2 garlic cloves, minced
4 wild-caught (fresh or frozen)
codfish filets
½ tsp. salt
½ tsp. dried thyme
4 eggs, beaten2 stalks scallions,
chopped
4 tbsp. black olives, sliced

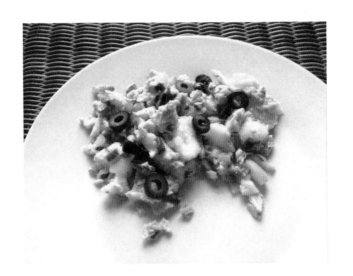

1. In a large skillet, heat 3 tbsp. butter over medium-high heat, and then add the onions, red bell pepper, and garlic. Cook for about 3 minutes until soft.
2. Add the codfish, salt, and thyme and turn the heat down to medium. Stir fry another 4 minutes breaking up the codfish into large chunks.
3. Pour in the eggs and continue to stir until the eggs are scrambled.
4. Garnish the dish with scallions and black olives.
5. Serve hot.

COOK'S NOTE
This delicious dish tastes very similar to the ackee and saltfish which is traditionally served for breakfast in Jamaica. Ackee fruit is cultivated in tropical regions and has a taste and texture very much like scrambled eggs. It is very hard to find in the US. Saltfish is simply a process of drying and salting cod for preservation.

NUTRITIONAL INFORMATION
Calories 299 Carbohydrate 5 g Fat 19 g Protein 27 g

COCONUT CRUSTED COD

The mild, delicate flavor of cod is enhanced with this crispy sweet coconut crust.

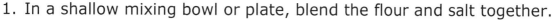

Serves 4

INGREDIENTS

6 tbsp. tapioca flour
¼ tsp. salt
1 egg, beaten
1 tbsp. honey
½ cup unsweetened coconut, shredded
3 tbsp. coconut oil
4 wild-caught (fresh or frozen) codfish filets, thawed and patted dry

1. In a shallow mixing bowl or plate, blend the flour and salt together.
2. In a separate shallow mixing bowl, beat the eggs, add the honey, and mix well.
3. Spread the coconut out on another plate.
4. In a large nonstick skillet, heat oil over medium-high heat.
5. Dredge the fish fillets in the flour, then the egg, and then press both sides into the shredded coconut.
6. Cook on one side to a light golden brown for about 3 minutes. Then turn and cook an additional 2-3 minutes. (If the filets are thick you might need to reduce the heat and cook another 2-3 minutes.)
7. Serve hot.

COOK'S NOTE

Excellent served with vegetable fried rice. Each serving provides 29% of your daily requirement for vitamin B6.

NUTRITIONAL INFORMATION

Calories 476 Carbohydrate 31 g Fat 30 g Protein 24 g

CREOLE-STYLE FISH

Spicy classic Creole-style seasonings bring a depth of flavor to simmered tomatoes and whitefish filets.

Serves 2

INGREDIENTS

2 tbsp. butter
2 tbsp. onion, chopped fine
2 garlic cloves, minced
2 tbsp. red bell pepper, chopped fine
2 tbsp. celery, chopped fine
2 cups tomato, chopped
¼ tsp. cayenne pepper
¼ tsp. red pepper flakes
¼ tsp. dried thyme
½ tsp. dried basil
¼ tsp. salt
2 fish filets (cod, mahi mahi or grouper) fresh, or thawed and patted dry
1 tsp. fresh lemon juice

1. In a large nonstick skillet, heat the butter over medium-high heat, and then add the onion, garlic, bell pepper, and celery. Cook for about 3 minutes until the vegetables are soft.
2. Add the tomatoes, cayenne pepper, pepper flakes, thyme, basil, and salt.
3. Allow it to come to a boil, and then reduce heat to medium and simmer for about 5 minutes. Stir occasionally.
4. Add the fish and lemon juice and continue to simmer another 6-7 minutes until the fish easily flakes.
5. Serve hot.

COOK'S NOTE
Any type of whitefish works with this spicy tomato-based Creole seasoned sauce. Pour it over rice for a delicious traditional southern Louisiana dish. Each serving provides 35% of your daily requirement for vitamin B6.

NUTRITIONAL INFORMATION

Calories 476 Carbohydrate 31 g Fat 30 g Protein 24 g

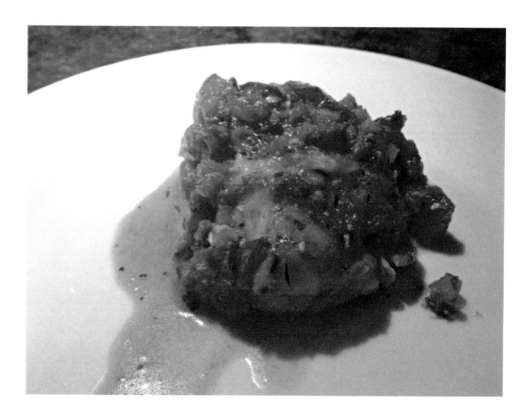

JERK CHICKEN PASTA

Chicken marinated in homemade jerk seasoning combine with pasta in this Jamaican-Italian fusion cuisine.

Serves 4

INGREDIENTS
1 cup water
½ cup white wine vinegar
1 sm. onion, chopped
1 sm. red or yellow bell pepper, chopped
3 Serrano peppers, chopped (or 1 tsp. cayenne pepper)
1 tbsp. allspice
1 tsp. dried ginger
½ tsp. salt
½ tsp. white or black pepper
½ tsp. dried thyme
¼ tsp. nutmeg
2 lg. boneless chicken breasts
3 cups Barilla Gluten-Free Penne or Shells (made with corn flour and rice flour), cooked and drained

Garlic Cream Cheese Sauce
¼ cup butter
2 garlic cloves, minced
8 oz. cream cheese
¼ tsp. salt
¼ tsp. white or black pepper
¼ tsp. dried oregano
¼ tsp. dried basil
½ cup water
Parmesan cheese (as desired)

1. In a small bowl, combine the first 11 ingredients and mix well.
2. Place the chicken breasts in a slow cooker and pour the mixture over the chicken.
3. Cook on low for 6-8 hours or on high for 3-4 hours.
4. Cook the pasta following package directions. As the pasta cooks, prepare the garlic cream sauce by heating the butter and garlic in a large nonstick skillet over medium-high heat for about 30 seconds.
5. Add the cheese, salt, pepper, oregano, basil, and water and reduce heat to a simmer, stirring often.
6. Remove the chicken breasts, shred, and set aside.
7. Pour the chicken jerk juices into the garlic cream sauce and blend them well.
8. Add the chicken and drained pasta to the skillet. Gently stir the dish to combine all ingredients.
9. Serve hot with a sprinkle of parmesan cheese on top.

COOK'S NOTE
There are a lot of ingredients and steps to this creamy pasta dish with spicy authentic jerk seasoning, but when it all comes together it's a very impressive meal rich in vitamin C, niacin, and B6.

Variation: Add fresh cooked asparagus to the meal.

NUTRITIONAL INFORMATION
Calories 585 Carbohydrate 37 g Fat 33 g Protein 34 g

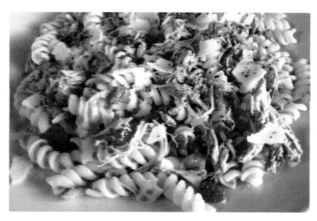

KENTUCKY-STYLE BOURBON CHICKEN

Sophisticated yet simple slow cooker bourbon chicken thighs are a traditional southern favorite.

Serves 4-6

INGREDIENTS

2 tbsp. butter
4-6 chicken thighs
1 tbsp. onion powder
¼ tsp. garlic powder
¼ cup white wine vinegar
1 tbsp. molasses
¼ cup honey
¼ cup bourbon
¼ cup maple syrup
½ tsp. dried ginger
¼ tsp. salt
¼ tsp. white pepper
1 tsp. red pepper flakes

1. Spread the butter around the bottom of the slow cooker.
2. Add the chicken.
3. Mix remaining ingredients in a bowl and pour over the chicken.
4. Cook on low for 6-8 hours or on high for 3-4 hours.
5. Serve hot.

COOK'S NOTE
Alcohol burns off during the cooking process and imparts a rich, robust flavor to the chicken thighs.

Variation: 2-3 chicken breasts can be substituted for the thighs.

NUTRITIONAL INFORMATION
Calories 291 Carbohydrate 21 g Fat 15 g Protein 11 g

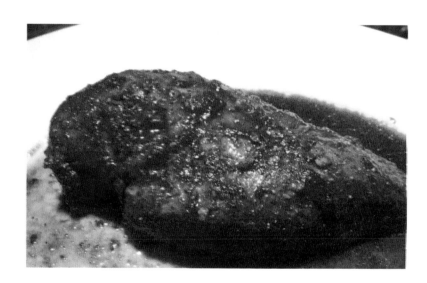

MEDITERRANEAN SKILLET FRITTATA

A variety of sautéed vegetables, eggs, and cheese create a one skillet meal with rich Italian flavor.

Serves 4
INGREDIENTS
1 tbsp. butter
⅓ cup red onion, diced
½ cup red or yellow bell pepper, diced
2 cloves garlic, minced
¼ cup button mushrooms, sliced
½ cup tomatoes, diced
½ cup zucchini, diced
1 tsp. dried Italian spice blend
¼ tsp. salt
½ tsp. crushed red pepper flakes
2 tbsp water
4 large eggs, beaten
½ cup olives, sliced
½ cup parmesan cheese
Black pepper (as desired)

1. In a large nonstick skillet, melt the butter over medium-high heat, and sauté the onions, peppers, garlic, and mushrooms until soft. (About 3 minutes.)
2. Stir in the tomatoes, zucchini, Italian seasoning, salt, red pepper flakes, and water. Cook another 3-4 minutes, stirring often.
3. In a medium-size bowl, beat the eggs and pour evenly across the top of the ingredients in the skillet.
4. Reduce the heat to medium-low and simmer for about 4-5 minutes without stirring.
5. At the end of the cooking time, lightly scrape the top to move any uncooked egg towards the sides of the skillet.

6. Top with olives and parmesan cheese and cook another minute to melt the cheese.
7. Remove from heat, slice like a pizza, and serve hot.

COOK'S NOTE
This quick and filling one skillet protein-packed meal is ideal for breakfast, lunch, or dinner.

NUTRITIONAL INFORMATION
Calories 276   Carbohydrate 9 g   Fat 19 g   Protein 18 g

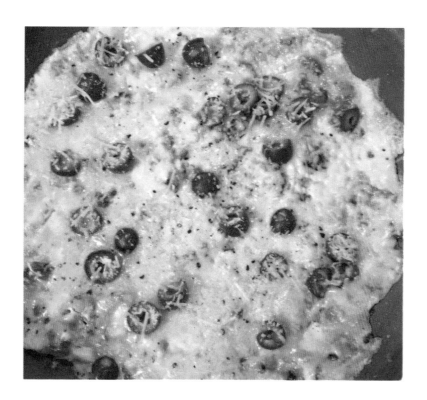

PIZZA CASSEROLE

This recipe is like a deep dish pizza with an amazing flourless crust.

SERVES 6-8
INGREDIENTS

CRUST
4 oz. cream cheese, softened
2 eggs
¼ tsp. dried Italian seasoning
¼ tsp. garlic powder
2 oz. parmesan cheese, shredded
8 oz. mozzarella cheese, shredded

TOPPINGS
1 tbsp. coconut oil
½ onion, diced
½ red or yellow pepper, diced
1 lb. ground grass-fed beef (or turkey, venison, bison)
5 roma tomatoes, chopped
1 tsp. olive oil
1 tsp. honey
1 garlic clove, chopped
1 tsp. dried Italian spices
4 oz. mozzarella cheese, shredded
4 oz. parmesan cheese, shredded

1. Preheat oven to 400 degrees.
2. In a medium-size bowl, blend the softened cream cheese with the eggs, Italian seasonings, and garlic until smooth and creamy.
3. Stir in the parmesan and mozzarella until it's all moistened.
4. Spread the crust mixture evenly in a well oiled 9x13 inch glass or ceramic baking dish
5. Bake 20-25 minutes until evenly browned.

6. In a large nonstick skillet or wok, heat the oil and stir-fry the diced onion and pepper, for about 3 minutes, until soft.
7. Add in the beef and cook until done.
8. Add in the tomato, olive oil, honey, garlic and Italian spice. Cook for about 3 more minutes, until the tomatoes are soft. (Add any additional pizza topping as desired.)
9. Spread the meat and vegetables over the cooked pizza crust and top with the mozzarella and parmesan cheeses.
10. Bake at 400 degrees for about 5 minutes or until the cheese is melted.
11. Let it stand for about 5 minutes; then cut and serve squares.

COOK'S NOTE
One serving of this hearty pizza supplies 52% of your daily requirement for vitamin B12 and 44% of your daily requirement for calcium.

NUTRITIONAL INFORMATION
Calories 457 Carbohydrate 8 g Fat 33 g Protein 34 g

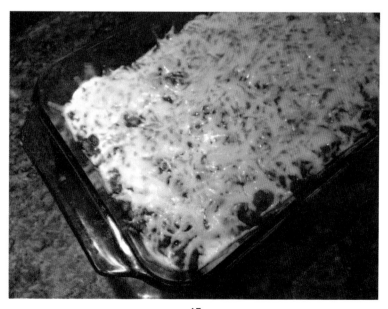

PUMPKIN CHILI

This rich, thick, and savory off-beat chili is packed with nutrition as well as flavor.

SERVES 4-6

INGREDIENTS
1 tbsp. coconut oil
1 onion, chopped
1 small red or yellow bell pepper, chopped
3 garlic cloves, minced
1 lb. ground grass-fed beef (or turkey, venison, bison)
3 cups tomatoes, diced
1 tsp. ground cumin
1 tsp. chili powder
½ tsp. cayenne pepper
1 tsp. dried basil
1 ½ cups black-eyed peas, purple hull peas or crowder peas. (12 oz. frozen pkg.)
2 cups water
2 cups pumpkin puree
Salt & pepper (as desired after cooking)
Optional toppings: raw pumpkin seeds, sour cream or shredded cheddar cheese

1. In a large saucepan, heat the coconut oil over medium-high heat, and cook the onion, bell pepper, and garlic. Cook for about 3 minutes, until soft.
2. Add the beef and break it up as it cooks. Cook until the meat is no longer pink.
3. Add diced tomatoes, cumin, chili powder, cayenne, basil, peas, water, and pumpkin to the beef mixture.
4. Bring to a boil and then reduce heat to medium-low. Cover and simmer 35 minutes. Sustain a rolling simmer and stir occasionally.
5. Serve in soup bowls with desired toppings.

COOK'S NOTE

No need to thaw the peas first. Add salt to recipe after it's cooked to avoid tough peas. Black-eyed peas are very low in oxalates making them the perfect "bean" for many recipes. They are especially high in potassium and zinc, which is important for the proper function of all cells.

NUTRITIONAL INFORMATION
Calories 581 Carbohydrate 65 g Fat 19 g   Protein 41 g

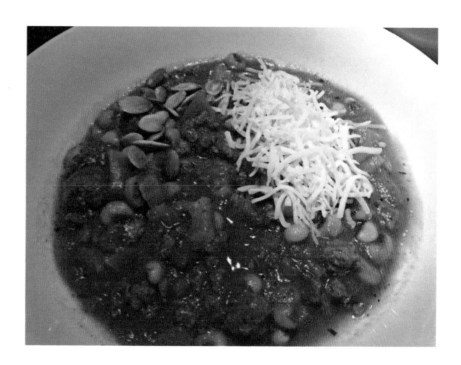

SLOW COOKER BEEF STEW

A full-bodied beef stew that is so simple yet incredibly delicious.

Serves 4
INGREDIENTS
1 tbsp. butter
1 lb. grass-fed beef stew meat, cut in 2 inch chunks
½ cup carrots, sliced thick
3 red skinned potatoes, peeled and quartered
1 onion, chopped
1 lg. tomato, chopped
1 ½ cup fresh or frozen green peas
1 tsp. salt
1 tsp. dried rosemary
½ tsp. thyme
½ tsp. pepper
2 tbsp. tapioca flour
½ cup red wine
2 cups chicken broth, bone broth or water

1. Spread the butter in the bottom of the slow cooker, add all of the ingredients, and mix well.
2. Cook on low for 8-10 hours or on high for 4-5 hours.
3. Serve in individual soup bowls.

COOK'S NOTE

It's unnecessary to be sure the liquid covers all of the ingredients in a slow cooker since the condensation continually rains down on the ingredients. This will be the easiest and tastiest beef stew you've ever cooked. Tapioca flour is a gluten-free thickening agent. It thickens at low temperatures and has a neutral taste, so it won't compete with other flavors.

NUTRITIONAL INFORMATION
Calories 571 Carbohydrate 65 g Fat 17 g Protein 35 g

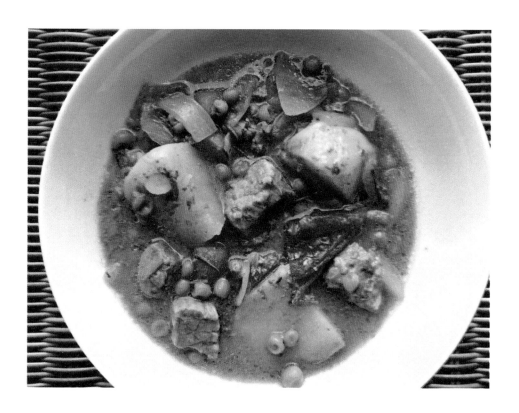

SLOW COOKER MUSTARD BARBECUE CHICKEN

This South Carolina style barbecue sauce adds a tangy sweet and spicy flavor to slow cooked chicken breasts.

SERVES 4

INGREDIENTS

1 tbsp. coconut oil
2 boneless chicken breasts
¼ cup white wine vinegar
¼ cup maple syrup
¼ cup water
1 tbsp. molasses
½ cup yellow mustard
3 garlic cloves, crushed
¼ tsp. paprika
¼ tsp. cayenne pepper
½ tsp. onion powder
¼ tsp. sea salt

1. Spread the oil in the bottom of the slow cooker and add the thawed chicken breasts.
2. In a bowl, mix remaining ingredients and pour over the chicken.
3. Cook on low 6-8 hours or on high for 4 hours.
4. Using two forks, shred the chicken and mix it with the sauce.
5. Serve over rice, on a bun, or with your favorite side dish.

COOK'S NOTE
This simple sauce is so delicious you will never be tempted to buy bottled barbecue sauce again.

NUTRITIONAL INFORMATION
Calories 213 Carbohydrate 10 g Fat 6 g Protein 29 g

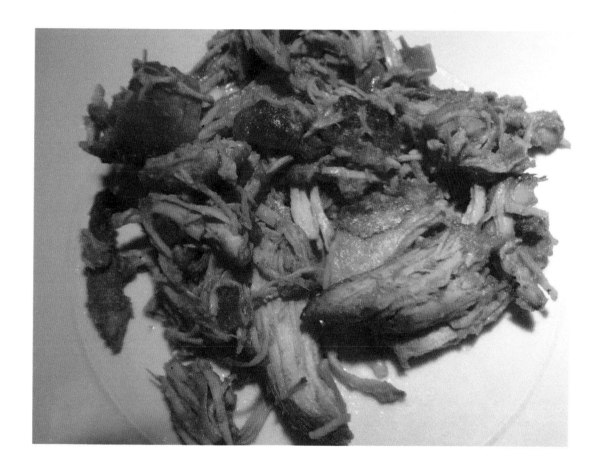

SLOW COOKER SANTA FE SOUP

The signature Tex-Mex flavors really come together in this rich warm soup.

Serves 4-6

INGREDIENTS

2 tbsp. extra virgin olive oil
1 medium onion, diced
3 garlic cloves, minced
5 medium tomatoes, chopped
½ red or yellow bell pepper, diced
¼ cup olives, sliced
1 cup corn
1 cup fresh or frozen black eyed peas (if using canned be sure to rinse and drain)
1 tsp. crushed red pepper flakes
1 tbsp. fresh cilantro, chopped
1 ½ tsp. cumin
1 tsp. salt
¼ tsp. pepper
¼ tsp. chili powder
3 cups chicken or bone broth
2 boneless chicken breasts
Cheddar cheese, shredded (as desired for topping)

1. Add all of the ingredients to the slow cooker and mix well.
2. Before serving use forks to pull apart the chicken breasts.
3. Serve in individual soup bowls and top with cheese as desired.

COOK'S NOTE
Black-eyed peas substitute for the typical black bean, which is high in oxalates.

NUTRITIONAL INFORMATION
Calories 500   Carbohydrate 54 g   Fat 13 g   Protein 46 g

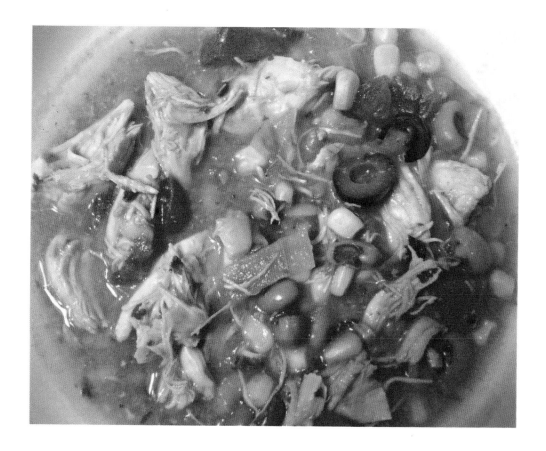

SLOW COOKER TAMALE PIE

A little tweak on the classic southwestern comfort food. This rich, warming meal tastes like the authentic Mexican tamale but without all of the work.

SERVES 6
INGREDIENTS
1 lb. ground grass-fed beef (or turkey, venison, bison)
½ medium onion, chopped
2 tsp. chili powder
1 tsp. cumin
3 medium tomatoes
2 garlic cloves
2 tsp. extra virgin olive oil
2 tbsp. Italian spices
1 tsp. honey
2-4 tbsp. olives, minced or sliced
2 cups corn
2 eggs, beaten
1 cup milk
2 tbsp. olive oil
1 ¼ cup yellow cornmeal, plain
1 tsp. baking powder
1 tsp. baking soda
½ tsp. salt
1 cup cheddar or monterey jack cheese, shredded

1. In a large mixing bowl, combine the ground beef, onion, chili powder, and cumin. Then press the meat mixture into the bottom of the slow cooker.
2. Puree the tomatoes, garlic, and olive oil in a blender or food processor. Then blend in the Italian spices and honey.
3. Pour the tomato puree over the meat.
4. Sprinkle the olives over the sauce and add the corn on top.
5. Mix the egg, milk, and oil together; then add the cornmeal, baking powder, baking soda, and salt. Mix and pour batter over the corn.

6. Cook on high for 4-5 hours.
7. Sprinkle the cheese on top and let it melt for 5 minutes before serving.

COOK'S NOTE
One serving of this flavor packed tamale pie delivers 48% of your daily requirement for B6, 32% of your daily requirement for potassium, and 24% of your daily requirement for magnesium.

NUTRITIONAL INFORMATION
Calories 407 Carbohydrate 40 g Fat 19 g Protein 22 g

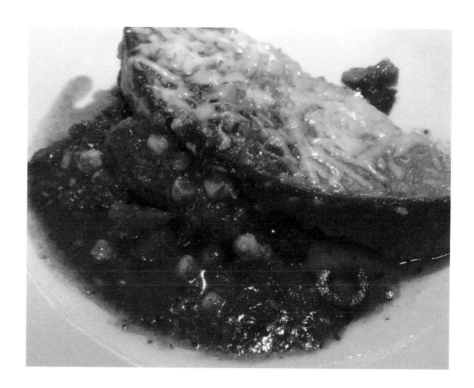

SOUTHWEST SALMON CAKES

The rich, velvety texture of avocado combined with wild Alaskan salmon and cumin gives these patties a slight southwest flair.

Serves 4-6
INGREDIENTS
½ avocado
1 egg
¼ tsp. white pepper
¼ tsp. dried dill
¼ tsp. cumin
2 tbsp. onion, diced
2 tbsp. red or yellow pepper, diced
14 oz. can wild Alaskan salmon, well drained
2-3 tbsp. coconut oil (for frying)
3 roma tomatoes, diced
1 cup corn
2 tsp. extra virgin olive oil
3 tbsp. plain whole milk yogurt
¼ tsp. dried basil
¼ tsp. garlic powder
Salt and pepper (as desired)

1. In a medium-size mixing bowl, mash the avocado and then blend it with the egg, pepper, dill, cumin, onion, and red pepper.
2. Stir in the salmon and mix well.
3. In a large nonstick skillet, heat the coconut oil over medium-high heat.
4. Form golf ball size balls then flatten a little after placing them in the heated oil. (Makes 8-10 patties.)
5. Cook patties until browned on one side, for about 4-5 minutes, then carefully turn and brown on the other side.

6. In a separate bowl, prepare the topping by combining the tomatoes, corn, oil, yogurt, basil, and garlic. Salt and pepper as desired.
7. Top the salmon cakes with a portion of the topping and serve.

COOK'S NOTE

Two top superfoods are teamed up in these incredibly tasty patties, which are just as delicious served without the salsa. One serving provides 100% of your daily requirement for vitamin D.

NUTRITIONAL INFORMATION
Calories 394 Carbohydrate 17 g Fat 26 g Protein 27 g

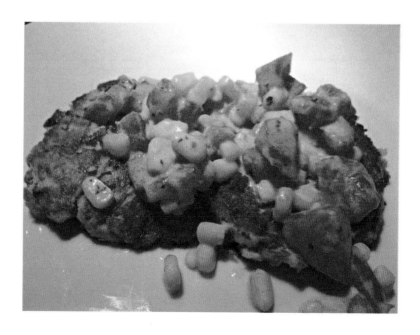

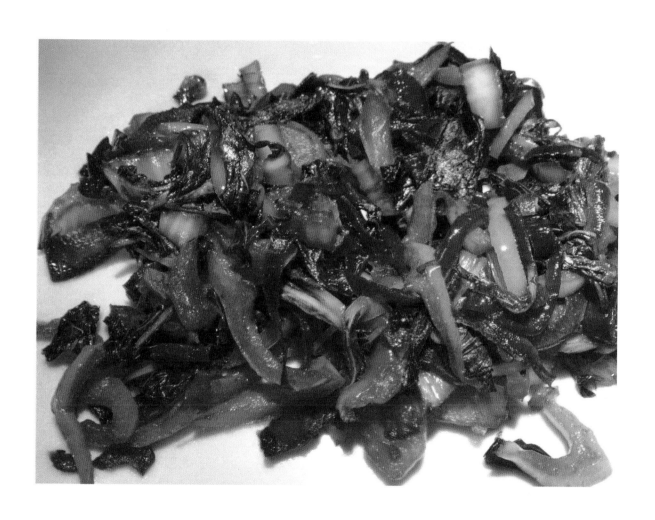

ARTICHOKES IN OLIVE SAUCE

The pungent flavor of garlic and the tangy taste of meaty black olives combine beautifully with artichoke hearts in this Italian side dish.

Serves 2-4
INGREDIENTS
¼ cup extra virgin olive oil
1 tbsp. onion, diced
3 garlic cloves, diced
1 tsp. tapioca flour
1 cup whole milk
½ cup black olives, sliced or minced
1 ½ cups artichoke hearts, thawed
1 tsp. lemon juice
2 tsp. Italian seasoning
¼ tsp. salt
½ tsp. white pepper

1. In a large nonstick skillet, heat the oil on medium heat and cook the onion and garlic until soft.
2. In a medium-size mixing bowl, whisk together the tapioca flour and milk.
3. Add the flour and milk blend to the skillet and continue to stir until thickened.
4. Add the olives, artichokes, lemon, Italian spices, salt, and pepper and continue to cook another 3-4 minutes.

COOK'S NOTE

Frozen artichoke hearts are used in this recipe to make it easier to prepare. Steaming and taking apart fresh artichokes to get to the hearts is a lot of work. Canned hearts tend to be mushy and, because of BPA toxicity, shouldn't be used, but the jarred version could be a replacement for frozen. Since the jarred version is usually in brine or marinated, rinse them well before using them in this recipe.

NUTRITIONAL INFORMATION
Calories 260 Carbohydrate 21 g Fat 19 g Protein 4 g

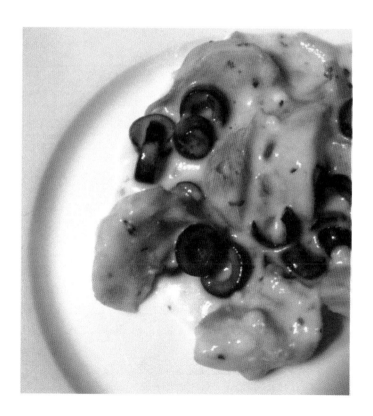

AVOCADO AND TOMATO SALAD

A simple summer salad with the flavorful combination of tomato and avocado.

Serves 4

INGREDIENTS

2 cups tomato, chopped
½ cup cucumber, chopped
2 tbsp. red onion, diced
2 tbsp. extra virgin olive oil
2 tsp. balsamic vinegar
¼ tsp. salt
3 garlic cloves, minced
1 tsp. dried basil
½ cup olives, sliced
2 avocados, peeled and chopped

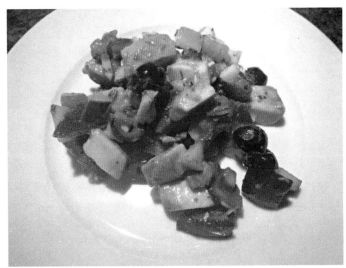

1. In a large mixing bowl, add all of the ingredients except the avocado and mix well.
2. Add the avocado and gently mix.
3. Let stand for about 5 minutes, and then gently mix again before serving.

COOK'S NOTE

A slight tweak on the traditional Greek salad introduces the rich and creamy texture of avocado as a replacement for lettuce and feta cheese. The many health benefits of avocado have made it a popular addition to any dish. This dish is an omega-3 powerhouse.

NUTRITIONAL INFORMATION
Calories 279 Carbohydrate 16 g Fat 25 g Protein 3 g

BOK CHOY STIR-FRY

Tender chopped bok choy with a touch of molasses gives this quick Chinese stir-fry a mildly sweet flavor.

Serves 4

INGREDIENTS

2 tbsp. coconut oil
½ medium onion, sliced thin
½ red or yellow pepper, sliced thin
2 garlic cloves, chopped
1 head bok choy, trimmed and chopped
½ tsp. dark molasses
¼ tsp. balsamic vinegar
¼ tsp. dried ginger
¼ tsp. red pepper flakes
¼ tsp. salt

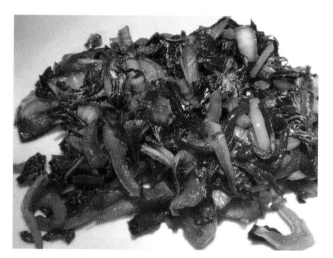

1. In a large nonstick skillet or wok, heat the oil over medium-high heat.
2. Add the onion, sliced pepper, and garlic.
3. Stir-fry for about 4 minutes until soft.
4. Add in the bok choy, molasses, vinegar, ginger, red pepper flakes, and salt.
5. Cook another 2-3 minutes until greens are wilted and stalks are crisp-tender.
6. Serve hot.

COOK'S NOTE

Bok choy is a type of Chinese cabbage that's very tender and rich in nutrients including omega-3, zinc, vitamin C, and vitamin K. The combination of balsamic vinegar, molasses, ginger and salt is a healthy alternative to soy sauce.

NUTRITIONAL INFORMATION
Calories 100 Carbohydrate 8 g Fat 7 g Protein 3 g

BUTTERED CABBAGE

A pure and simple side dish loaded with a sweet buttery flavor.

Serves 4
INGREDIENTS
½ large green or purple head of cabbage
½ cup butter
¼ tsp. salt
⅛ tsp. pepper

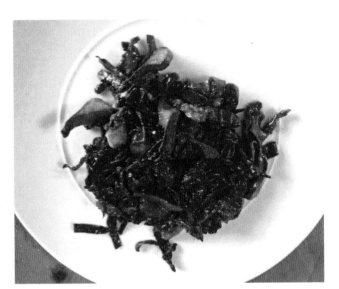

1. Remove outer leaves, cut in half, and remove the core of the cabbage.
2. Halve the sections again and slice the cabbage into thin shreds.
3. In a large nonstick skillet, melt the butter over medium-heat, and then add the cabbage, salt, and pepper.
4. Cook for about 5 minutes, stirring occasionally, and then cover.
5. Turn the heat down to medium-low and continue to cook for about 5 minutes more or until the cabbage is tender.
6. Serve hot.

COOK'S NOTE
A great accompaniment to pork, beef, or chicken. One serving of this buttery cabbage supplies 100% of your vitamin K requirements.

NUTRITIONAL INFORMATION
Calories 232 Carbohydrate 7 g Fat 23 g Protein 2 g

CHEESY ASPARAGUS CAKES

Fresh asparagus teams up with parmesan cheese in these delicious pan fried cakes.

Serves 6

INGREDIENTS

Water, lightly salted (for boiling)
2 cups asparagus, cut in 1 inch pieces.
¼ tsp. onion powder
¼ tsp. dried thyme
1 egg, beaten
½ cup parmesan cheese, shredded
¼ cup rice flour
1 tbsp. butter

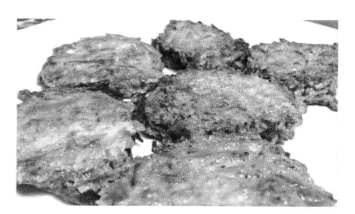

1. Bring ½ inch salted water to a boil in a large skillet; then add the asparagus.
2. Cook the asparagus for about 7 minutes until asparagus is tender.
3. Drain and transfer to a medium-size mixing bowl.
4. Crush the asparagus pieces and add the onion, thyme, egg, parmesan, and rice flour. Mix well.
5. In a large nonstick skillet, heat the butter over medium heat.
6. Drop large spoonfuls of the asparagus mixture into the heated butter. Press each with the back of a spoon to flatten into patties and fry about 2-3 minutes on each side until golden brown.
7. Transfer to a serving dish and continue with the remaining mixture. Makes 10-12 cakes. (You may need to turn the heat down to medium-low and add more butter for the second batch.)

COOK'S NOTE

Asparagus doesn't have to be completely pureed in this recipe. You want to have some texture in each cheesy bite of these fried cakes.

NUTRITIONAL INFORMATION
Calories 112 Carbohydrate 13 g Fat 5 g Protein 5 g

CURRIED CAULIFLOWER

The Indian spices and tomato combination adds an exotic flavor and color to cauliflower.

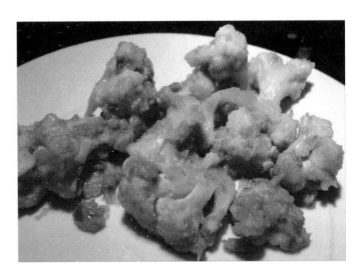

SERVES 4
INGREDIENTS
1 onion, diced
2 garlic cloves, minced
1 tomato, chopped
1 tsp. dried basil
1 ½ tsp. curry powder
½ tsp. dried ginger or 1 ½ tbsp. fresh minced ginger
½ tsp. red pepper flakes
1 tbsp. butter
1 cup water
½ medium head cauliflower florets, cut bite size

1. In a medium-size saucepan, bring the onion, garlic, tomato, basil, curry powder, ginger, red pepper flakes, butter and water to a boil.
2. Reduce heat to medium, add the cauliflower florets, and continue to simmer for about 12 minutes. Stir occasionally and check for tenderness.
3. Serve hot.

COOK'S NOTE
A perfect, spicy side dish for fish or chicken but can also be served as a vegetarian main dish when served with rice or lentils.

NUTRITIONAL INFORMATION
Calories 62 Carbohydrate 8 g Fat 3 g Protein 2 g

MARINATED VEGETABLE SALAD

Flavorful crisp-tender vegetables in a tangy sweet marinade.

Serves 4
INGREDIENTS

1 ½ cups fresh asparagus, cut in 1 inch pieces
2 cups cauliflower florets cut in bite size pieces
¼ cup small red onion, diced
2 tbsp. extra virgin olive oil
2 tbsp. white wine vinegar or lemon juice
1 tsp. honey
¼ tsp. dried basil
¼ tsp. salt

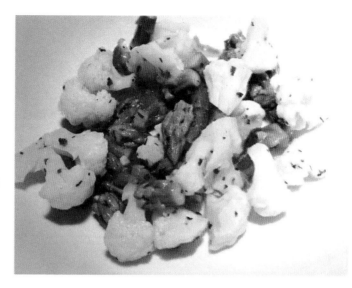

1. In a small saucepan, cover the asparagus, cauliflower, and onion with water and bring to a boil.
2. Reduce heat to a simmer for 3 minutes.
3. While the vegetables cook combine the olive oil, wine vinegar or lemon juice, honey, basil, and salt in a large bowl.
4. Drain the vegetables and add to the marinade.
5. Mix well and chill for about an hour. Toss occasionally and toss again before serving.

COOK'S NOTE
Serve as a salad, side dish, or light refreshing vegetarian dinner.

NUTRITIONAL INFORMATION
Calories 100 Carbohydrate 9 g Fat 7 g Protein 2 g

MASHED POTATOES WITH VEGETABLE GRAVY
Rich, flavorful potatoes topped with a smooth vegetable gravy puree.

Serves 6
INGREDIENTS
2 tbsp. butter
6 potatoes, peeled and halved lengthwise
2 medium onions, chopped
1 small red or yellow pepper, chopped
3 garlic cloves, chopped
2 zucchini squash, chopped
½ head fresh cauliflower florets, cut bite size
½ tsp. salt
¼ tsp. white pepper
¼ tsp. sage
¼ tsp. dried rosemary
⅓ cup water
¼ cup whole milk

1. Spread the butter in the bottom of the slow cooker.
2. Place the potatoes in the bottom making sure none touch the side of the slow cooker.
3. Add the onion, pepper, garlic, zucchini, cauliflower, salt, pepper, sage, dried rosemary, and water to a large bowl and mix well.
4. Add the mixed vegetables to the slow cooker and cook on low for 6-8 hours or on high for 3-4 hours.
5. When cooking time is over transfer 8 or 9 potato halves to a medium-size mixing bowl, add the milk, and mash to desired consistency.
6. Add the remaining slow cooker ingredients to a blender and blend on high speed until smooth and creamy.
7. Serve the mashed potatoes with desired amount of vegetable gravy on top.

COOK'S NOTE

These fully cooked vegetables make surprisingly rich, flavorful gravy without the use of any thickening agent. This recipe makes a large amount of gravy that can be served over any accompanied meat. It also freezes well for future use.

NUTRITIONAL INFORMATION
Calories 347 Carbohydrate 70 g Fat 5 g Protein 10 g

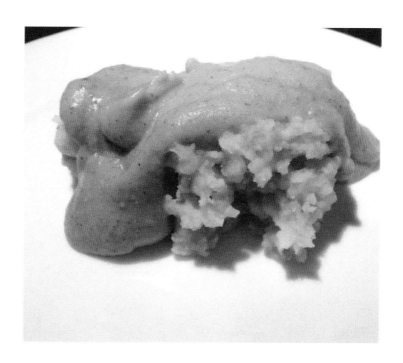

RATATOUILLE

A combination of fresh summer produce slow cooked to a rich flavorful stew.

Serves 4
INGREDIENTS
3 tomatoes, quartered
2 zucchini, sliced thick
2 yellow squash, sliced thick
1 cup cauliflower florets
1 red or yellow bell pepper, chopped
1 medium onion, chopped
½ cup olives, halved or sliced
4 tbsp. extra virgin olive oil
4 garlic cloves, diced
1 tsp. fresh dried basil
½ tsp. dried thyme
¼ tsp. salt
⅛ tsp. pepper
½ cup parmesan cheese, grated (optional)

1. Combine all of the ingredients except the parmesan cheese in a slow cooker and mix well.
2. Cook on low heat for 6-8 hours or on high for 3-4 hours.
3. Serve hot.

COOK'S NOTE

The traditional French ratatouille is usually prepared as a thick stew with each vegetable sautéed individually and then combined and baked. This slow cooker version is equally terrific in taste and much simpler to prepare. Serve it as a side dish to any meat or pour it over rice or eggs and top with cheese for a main dish.

NUTRITIONAL INFORMATION
Calories 227 Carbohydrate 18 g Fat 17 g Protein 5 g

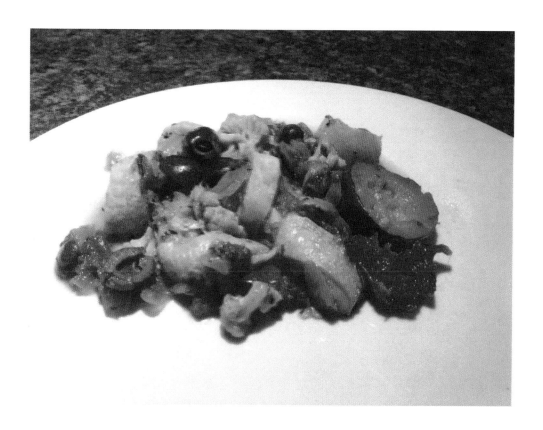

SAUTÉED BRUSSELS SPROUTS

These tiny cabbages simply sautéed with tomato and onion create a flavorful one skillet vegetarian dish or can be paired with fish or chicken.

Serves 4
INGREDIENTS
1 tbsp. butter
2 cloves garlic, chopped
½ onion, chopped
2 medium tomatoes, chopped
¼ tsp. salt
½ tsp. red pepper flakes
½ tsp. dried thyme
1 tsp. dried basil
1 ½ cups fresh or frozen Brussels sprouts, thawed and halved
½ cup water
Parmesan cheese (as desired)

1. In a large nonstick skillet, heat the butter over medium heat, and then add the garlic and onion. Cook for about 3 minutes until soft.
2. Add the tomatoes, salt, pepper flakes, thyme, and basil. Continue to cook another 2 minutes until tomatoes are tender.
3. Add the halved Brussels sprouts and water and continue to cook over medium heat another 15 minutes with occasional stirring.
4. Serve hot topped with parmesan as desired.

COOK'S NOTE

Brussels sprouts are related to a wild variety of cabbage that originated near the Mediterranean. They are named after the city of Brussels in Belgium. Brussels sprouts are high in protein, low in carbohydrate, and are high in vitamins C, K, and A.

NUTRITIONAL INFORMATION

Calories 78 Carbohydrate 11 g Fat 3 g Protein 4 g

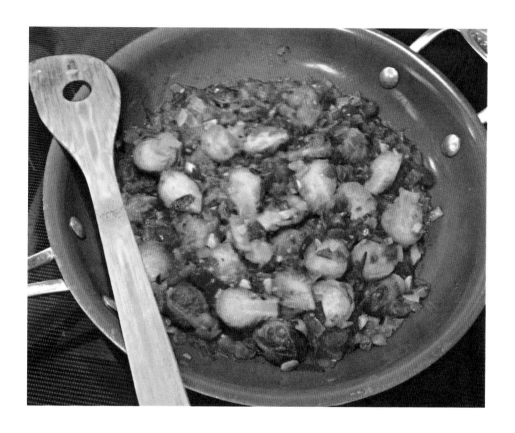

SAVORY SAVOY SLAW

A tender, tangy, and fresh tasting slaw with a hint of creaminess to bind it together.

Serves 4-6

INGREDIENTS

½ head savoy cabbage
¼ cup white wine vinegar
¼ cup honey
2 tbsp. plain whole milk yogurt
2 tbsp. extra virgin olive oil
½ tsp. salt
¼ tsp. white pepper
¼ tsp. crushed red pepper flakes

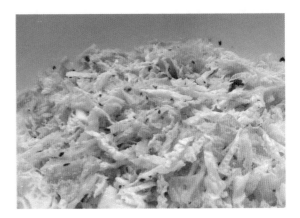

1. Slice the cabbage in half through the core. Cut a v-shaped notch around the white core and discard the core. Slice lengthwise into quarters and thinly slice each quarter crosswise into strips.
2. In a medium-size mixing bowl, whisk together the wine vinegar, honey, yogurt, oil, salt, and peppers.
3. Pour the dressing over the shredded cabbage. Mix well.
4. Allow to sit for about 15 minutes but stir occasionally to meld the flavors during this time.
5. Can be served room temperature or chilled.

COOK'S NOTE

Any cabbage can be used in this recipe. Green is the most common and red cabbage will give the slaw a more peppery flavor. Savoy cabbage has the most delicate flavor and a little less crunch. If green or red cabbage is used, add another ¼ tsp. salt and let it sit at least 30 minutes before serving.

NUTRITIONAL INFORMATION
Calories 112 Carbohydrate 12 g Fat 7 g Protein 0 g

SLOW COOKER INDIAN LENTILS

A fragrant traditional Indian side dish of protein rich lentils spiced up with curry, cumin, and cayenne.

Serves 4-6

INGREDIENTS

2 cups green or yellow lentils
2 tbsp. coconut oil
½ tsp. curry powder
½ tsp. dry mustard
¼ tsp. cumin
½ tsp. cayenne pepper
¼ tsp. dried ginger
3 cloves garlic, chopped
1 small onion, chopped
2 medium tomatoes, chopped
4 cups chicken or bone broth
Salt (as desired)*

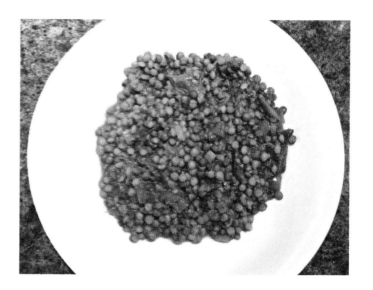

1. Sort and rinse the lentils under warm water.
2. Spread the oil over the bottom of the slow cooker.
3. Add all ingredients to the slow cooker and mix well.
4. Cover and cook on low for 6-8 hours or on high for 3-4 hours.
5. Serve hot.

COOK'S NOTE

Unlike most dried beans or legumes, lentils require no soaking before cooking. Lentils are a good source of magnesium and fiber. These hearty lentils may be served with rice or any meat, poultry, or fish.
*Salt will toughen lentils if added during the cooking time, so it's best to salt them after they are cooked.

NUTRITIONAL INFORMATION
Calories 461 Carbohydrate 64 g Fat 9 g Protein 31 g

TEX-MEX SPAGHETTI SQUASH

Silky spaghetti squash topped with seasoned corn, melted cheese, and diced avocado.

Serves 6-8
INGREDIENTS
1 spaghetti squash, cooked*
1 cup cheddar, shredded and divided
2 tbsp. butter
1 medium onion, chopped
1 cup corn
1 medium tomato, diced
½ tsp. chili powder
1 tsp. cumin
¼ tsp. garlic powder
¼ tsp. salt
¼ tsp. pepper

1. Slice the cooked squash in half and remove the peeling and the seeds.
2. Line the bottom of a 9x13 casserole dish with the squash and press it down.
3. Top the squash with half of the cheddar cheese.
4. In a large nonstick skillet, melt the butter over medium-high heat and cook the onion for about 3 minutes until soft.
5. Add the corn and stir-fry about 2 minutes (if using frozen corn cook an extra minute) Then add the tomato and cook 1 more minute.
6. Pour the cooked onion, corn, and tomato over the squash, spread it out evenly, and season with chili powder, cumin, salt, and pepper.
7. Top with the remaining cheese and place the dish under the broiler for about 2-3 minutes to melt the cheese.
8. Serve hot.

COOK'S NOTE

*The simplest way to have cooked squash already prepared for this dinner is to put it in the slow cooker in the morning. Puncture it a few times with a sharp knife and cook it on low for 6-8 hours.

NUTRITIONAL INFORMATION

Calories 212 Carbohydrate 23 g Fat 11 g Protein 8 g

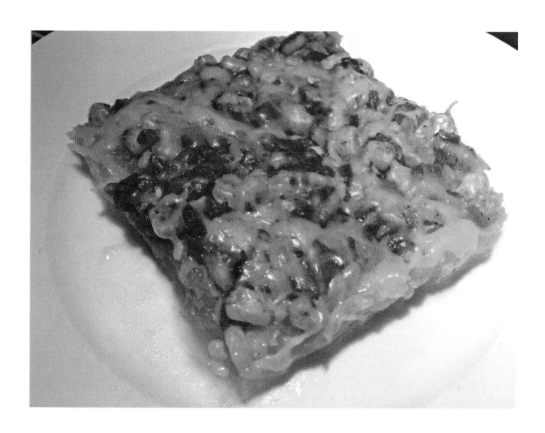

VEGETABLE FRIED RICE

Each bite of this simple stir-fried rice offers a colorful mix of flavors.

Serves 4-6
INGREDIENTS
2 tbsp. coconut oil
1 red onion, chopped
3 garlic cloves, minced
¼ cup carrot, chopped
¼ cup yellow or red bell pepper, chopped
½ cup cabbage, chopped, (any type cabbage works well)
½ cup green peas, (frozen is fine)
1 tbsp. water
1 tsp. balsamic vinegar
1 tsp. dark molasses
¼ tsp. ginger
2 eggs, beaten
2 cups cooked rice
½ tsp. salt
¼ tsp. pepper

1. In a large nonstick skillet or wok, heat the oil over high heat
2. Add the onion, garlic, carrot, and bell pepper and stir fry for about 3 minutes until soft.
3. Stir in the cabbage, peas, water, vinegar, molasses, and ginger. Cook for 3 minutes, stirring constantly.
4. Add the beaten eggs and continue to stir-fry until the eggs are cooked.
5. Add the cooked rice and stir-fry until mixed thoroughly with the vegetables.
6. Season with salt and pepper and serve hot.

COOK'S NOTE

If you desire a less sticky rice, cook the rice ahead of time and refrigerate. Additional time will be needed to stir-fry until the dish is hot. The traditional soy sauce or tamari are not needed to enjoy fried rice dishes. Both are made from soybeans which are high in oxalates and unless bought organic are often genetically modified. A healthy alternative to soy sauce is the combination of balsamic vinegar, molasses, ginger, and salt.

NUTRITIONAL INFORMATION
Calories 311 Carbohydrate 49 g Fat 9 g Protein 8 g

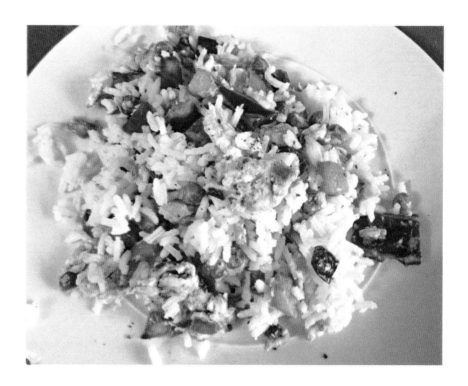

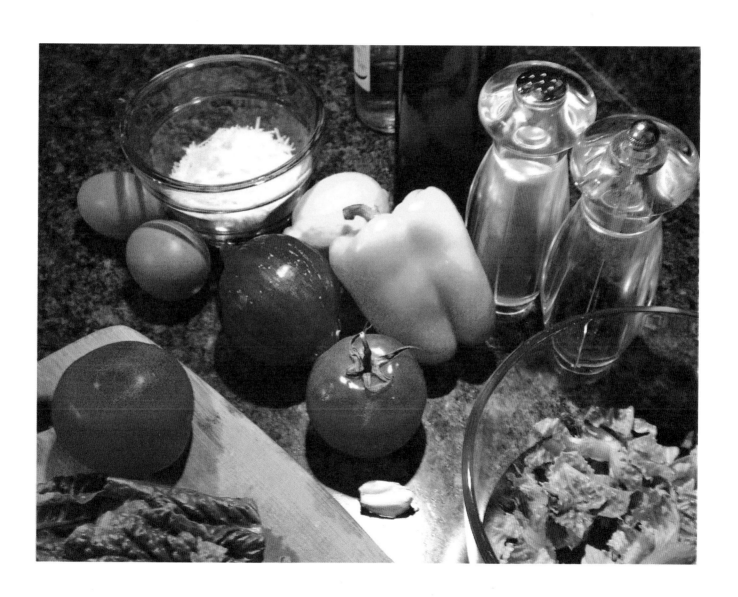

BALSAMIC DRESSING

¾ cup extra virgin olive oil
¼ cup balsamic vinegar
1 tbsp. honey

Place all of the ingredients in a jar, cover tightly, and shake. Keep refrigerated up to 10 days.

CAESAR DRESSING

½ cup extra virgin olive oil
1 egg
3 garlic cloves
2 tbsp. white wine vinegar
1 tsp. dry mustard
1 tsp. molasses
¼ cup parmesan cheese
4-5 anchovies
Black pepper (as desired)

Add all of the ingredients to a blender and process for 30 seconds until the mixture is smooth. Keep refrigerated up to one week. Bring to room temperature and shake or whisk well before serving.

HONEY MUSTARD DRESSING

½ cup mustard
¼ cup honey
¼ cup plain whole milk yogurt
1 tbsp. extra virgin olive oil
1 tbsp. white wine vinegar

Place all of the ingredients in a jar, cover tightly, and shake. Keep refrigerated up to one week. Bring to room temperature and shake well before serving.

ITALIAN DRESSING

1 cup extra virgin olive oil
½ cup white wine vinegar
¼ tsp. garlic powder
¼ tsp. dried rosemary
¼ tsp. dried oregano
¼ tsp. dried basil

Place all of the ingredients in a jar, cover tightly, and shake. Allow to sit at least 30 minutes to meld the ingredients. Keep refrigerated up to 10 days. Bring to room temperature and shake well before serving.

RANCH DRESSING

½ cup butter
½ tsp, garlic powder
½ tsp. chives
¼ tsp. onion powder
¼ tsp. parsley
¼ tsp. dill
1 cup plain whole milk yogurt

Melt the butter, whisk in all of the seasonings, and mix in the yogurt. Allow to sit at least 20 minutes to meld the ingredients. Keep refrigerated up to one week. Bring to room temperature and shake well before serving.

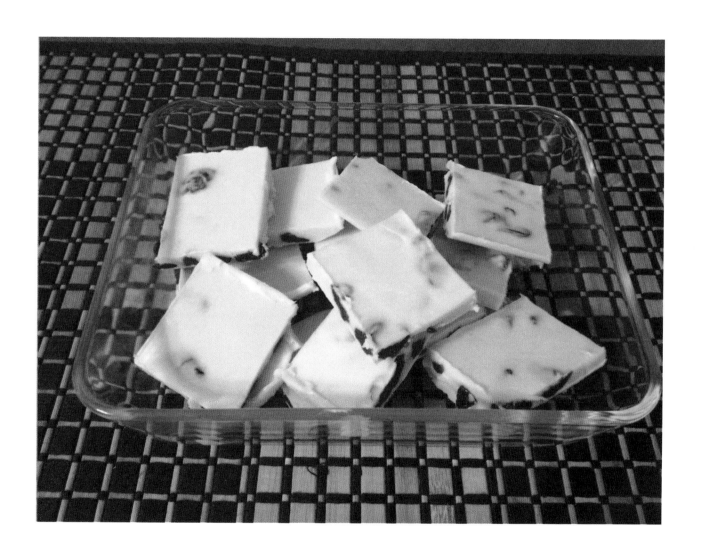

COCONUT CAKE

A moist, protein and fiber rich cake made with coconut flour. It's just as healthy as it is delicious.

Serves 10-12
INGREDIENTS
6 tbsp. coconut flour
½ tsp. baking soda
¼ tsp. salt
5 eggs
½ cup maple syrup
2 tsp. vanilla
½ cup coconut oil, melted
½ cup unsweetened coconut, shredded

Frosting
8 oz. cream cheese, softened
2 tbsp. butter, melted
¼ cup plain whole milk yogurt
1 tsp. vanilla
1 cup maple syrup
1 cup unsweetened coconut, shredded

1. Preheat oven to 325 degrees.
2. Oil a 9x13 inch glass or ceramic baking dish.
3. Mix coconut flour, baking soda, and salt in a medium-size bowl.
4. In a separate bowl, add the eggs, syrup, vanilla, and coconut oil.
5. Pour the wet ingredients into the dry and mix well using an electric blender on the lowest speed until very smooth.
6. Stir in the shredded coconut and pour the batter into the baking dish. Spread evenly.
7. Bake 35 minutes.

8. Use an electric blender to blend all of the frosting ingredients until smooth. Then add 1 cup of coconut flakes and mix well with a spoon.
9. Allow the cake to cool, for about 30 minutes, before topping it with frosting.

COOK'S NOTE
It is easy to have variations of this cake. Simply replace the shredded coconut with fresh chopped strawberries or pineapple in both the cake and the frosting. The taste and texture is similar to a classic yellow cake.

NUTRITIONAL INFORMATION
Calories 651 Carbohydrate 44 g Fat 52 g Protein 7 g

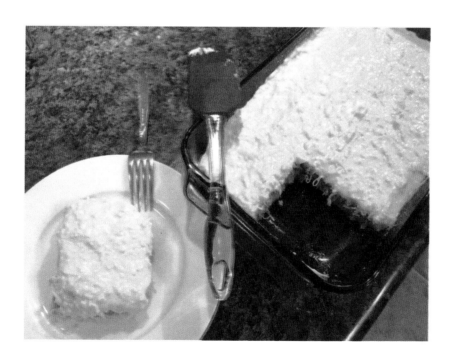

COCONUT CREAM SNOWBALLS

This creamy, crunchy, no bake coconut dessert is an all natural delight.

Serves 6
INGREDIENTS
8 oz. cream cheese, softened
3 tbsp. honey
½ tsp. vanilla
½ tsp. coconut flour
1 cup unsweetened coconut, shredded

1. Combine the cream cheese, honey, vanilla and flour. Blend well.
2. Spread some shredded coconut out on a plate, drop a spoonful of batter onto the plate, and use both hands to shape the snowball as you coat with shredded coconut. Toss from hand to hand to remove excess coconut. Makes 12-14.
3. Repeat the process and add shredded coconut to the plate when needed.
4. Refrigerate for an hour before serving.

COOK'S NOTE
Eating healthy through the holidays can be a real challenge, but these fast and fabulous coconut cream snowballs satisfy that sweet craving without sacrificing your health.

NUTRITIONAL INFORMATION
Calories 438 Carbohydrate 20 g Fat 40 g Protein 6 g

EASY CHEESECAKE

A moist and delicious cheesecake with a buttery, cookie-like, coconut flour crust.

Serves 8
INGREDIENTS
Crust
¾ cup coconut flour
¼ tsp. salt
½ cup butter, melted
1 tbsp. and ½ cup honey
2 eggs
Filing
4 eggs
16 oz. cream cheese, softened
1 tsp. vanilla
1½ cups plain whole milk yogurt

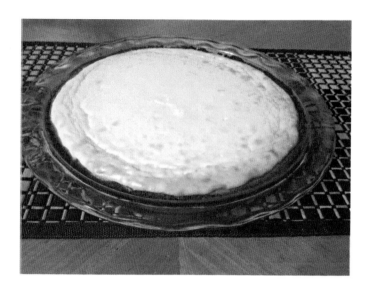

1. Preheat oven to 400 degrees.
2. In a large mixing bowl, mix the coconut flour with the salt and set aside.
3. In a separate mixing bowl, blend the butter, 1 tbsp. honey, and 2 eggs.
4. Add the wet ingredients to the dry and mix well.
5. Oil a 10 inch deep dish glass pie plate and press the crust mixture across the bottom and halfway up the sides of the pie dish. Bake 8 minutes.
6. Remove the crust and turn the oven down to 350 degrees.
7. Add the remaining (½ cup) honey, eggs, cream cheese, vanilla, and yogurt to a bowl and blend on low speed until smooth. Pour it into the pie crust and bake about 55 minutes.
8. Chill an hour or two before serving.

COOK'S NOTE
The coconut flour crust will darken quite a bit and give it a nutty taste.

NUTRITIONAL INFORMATION
Calories 556 Carbohydrate 23 g Fat 49 g Protein 11 g

FRUITCAKE

This gluten-free fruitcake has a lighter texture but similar taste when compared to the traditional fruitcake.

Serves 8-10
INGREDIENTS
7 tbsp. coconut flour
½ tsp. baking soda
1 tsp. baking powder
¼ tsp. salt
1 tsp. instant coffee grounds
6 tbsp. water
4 eggs
½ cup maple syrup
1 tsp. vanilla
½ tsp. nutmeg
¼ tsp. ginger
½ cup coconut oil, melted
¼ cup unsweetened coconut, shredded
½ cup raisins
½ cup raw pumpkin seeds
½ cup dried pineapple, chopped
½ cup dried cherries, chopped

1. Preheat oven to 350 degrees.
2. Oil a 6x9 loaf pan.
3. Mix coconut flour, baking soda, baking powder, and salt in a medium-size bowl and set aside.
4. In a separate bowl, mix coffee and water first and then add in the eggs, syrup, vanilla, nutmeg, ginger, and coconut oil.
5. Pour the wet ingredients into the dry and mix well using an electric blender until very smooth.
6. Stir in the shredded coconut, raisins, pumpkin seeds, pineapple, and cherries and pour the mix into the baking dish.

7. Bake 40 minutes.
8. Allow to cool before removing from pan.

COOK'S NOTE

Fruitcake dates back to the middle ages. Recipes have varied greatly throughout the ages depending on what was available. This variation replaces grain flour with coconut flour and eliminates the alcohol which was traditionally used to preserve the fruitcake. Fruitcakes are enjoyed throughout the year in most countries today, but in the US it's mainly served during the Christmas holidays. However, this tasty variation may have you preparing it throughout the year.

NUTRITIONAL INFORMATION
Calories 380 Carbohydrate 26 g Fat 6 g Protein 3 g

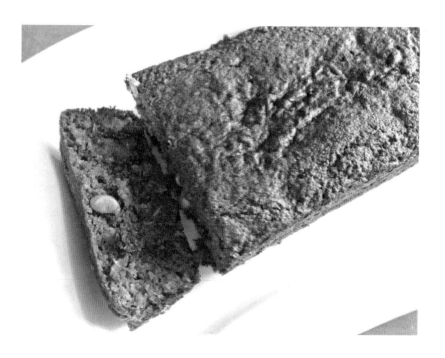

WHITE CHOCOLATE CHERRY SQUARES

A simple yet elegant looking dessert of chewy cherries in sweet white chocolate.

Serves 8-10

INGREDIENTS

1/3 cup coconut oil
2 cups white chocolate chips
1 ½ tsp. vanilla
A pinch of salt
1 cup dried cherries

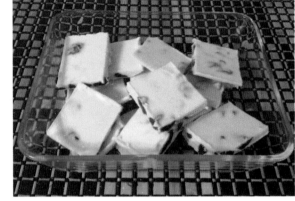

1. In a medium-size saucepan, melt the coconut oil and chocolate chips over medium-high heat stirring constantly.
2. Remove from heat and blend in the vanilla, salt, and cherries.
3. Pour into an oiled 9x13 glass baking dish.
4. Refrigerate about an hour before cutting and serving.

COOK'S NOTE

Continually dip a sharp knife in a glass of hot water to cut the squares. Cherries are packed with antioxidants and offer many health benefits.

NUTRITIONAL INFORMATION
Calories 314 Carbohydrate 26 g Fat 23 g Protein 3 g

WHITE CHOCOLATE CHIP COOKIES

America's favorite cookie made gluten-free with coconut flour and made low in oxalates by using white chocolate chips. A light, textured cookie that is simple yet divine.

Makes 16-18
INGREDIENTS
¼ cup butter, melted
¼ cup honey
2 eggs
½ tsp. vanilla
½ tsp. baking soda
¼ tsp. salt
½ cup coconut flour
¾ cup white chocolate chips

1. Preheat oven to 350 degrees.
2. Cover a large baking sheet with parchment paper.
3. In a medium-size bowl, mix the melted butter with the honey until smooth; then add in the eggs, vanilla, baking soda, and salt. Mix well.
4. Blend in the coconut flour and allow to stand about 1 minute as the coconut flour absorbs the liquid ingredients. Then mix in the white chocolate chips.
5. Shape spoonfuls into balls and place on the baking sheet. Makes 16-18 cookies.
6. Using a fork, press down each cookie to the desired size. (Cookies will not spread out or rise much.)
7. Cook 15-16 minutes. The outside of the cookie should be a golden brown color.
8. Slide the parchment paper off onto a counter and cool for 10 minutes before removing to a serving dish.

COOK'S NOTE
Using honey with coconut flour in a cookie recipe gives the perfect dough consistency for an excellent chewy cookie. These are a dream come true for the gluten intolerant and low-oxalate dieter.

NUTRITIONAL INFORMATION
Calories 293 Carbohydrate 22 g Fat 22 g Protein 4 g

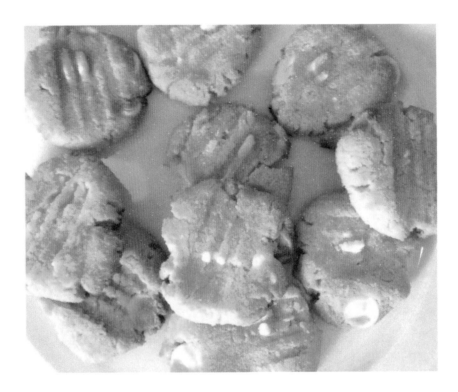

WHITE CHOCOLATE MOUNDS

Melt in your mouth white chocolate with a sweet gooey, chewy, coconut center.

Serves 6
INGREDIENTS
2 cups unsweetened coconut, shredded
¼ cup coconut oil, melted
½ cup honey
1 tsp. vanilla
½ cup plain whole milk yogurt
12 oz. white chocolate chips

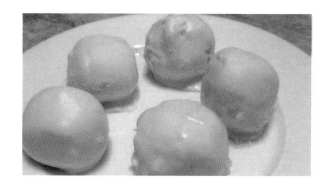

1. In a large mixing bowl, combine the coconut, oil, honey, vanilla, and yogurt.
2. Form 1 ½ inch balls (12-14) of coconut mix and place in the freezer for 15 minutes.
3. Melt the chocolate using a double broiler. (Make your own double broiler by selecting a small saucepan and a bowl that will fit over it without falling inside. The bowl should dip partially inside the saucepan. Add 1 inch of water to the small saucepan, and bring it to a light boil over medium-high heat. Add the chocolate to the small bowl on top. Stir gently and continuously until melted. Carefully remove the bowl of melted chocolate and transfer to a heat-safe surface.)
4. Using 2 forks, dip one ball at a time into the melted chocolate and place on a baking sheet or on a sheet of parchment paper.
5. Let chocolate set before serving.

COOK'S NOTE
These delicious candies are not sugar-free, but they are a much healthier alternative to processed store bought candy.

NUTRITIONAL INFORMATION
Calories 918 Carbohydrate 60 g Fat 76 g Protein 9 g

Melinda Keen is an author, middle school teacher, and certified nutrition consultant. Her previous works include *Mud in My Heart* (2007) a young adult novel and *Low Oxalate Fresh and Fast Cookbook* (2015). Her first cookbook, Low *Oxalate Fresh and Fast Cookbook,* grew out of her love of cooking and the desire to help others prepare a variety of fresh and healthy meals low in oxalates. Her experience with chronic illness and research on the potential ill effects of oxalates in foods led her to evaluate and rework her recipes which transformed her own life and health. A low-oxalate diet is a meal plan that is low in oxalates to help heal symptoms of bladder pain, kidney stones, irritable bowel syndrome, fibromyalgia, and pain associated with oxalate stone formation in other parts of the body. It is a prevention diet often recommended for kidney stone issues. The *Low Oxalate Fresh and Fast Cookbook* contains healthy, delicious recipes that include casseroles, pastas, soups, stir-fries, and slow cooker meals. The book contains a collection of meals that are perfect for the cook who wants home-cooked, nutritious, fresh food fast. Each recipe includes mouthwatering photography, useful cook's tips, and nutritional information.

Melinda is a wife, mother, grandmother, nutritionist, and educator presently living in Tennessee.

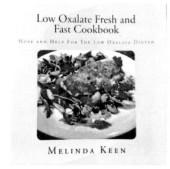

Low Oxalate Fresh and Fast Cookbook
ISBN 13: 978-1511675918

Healthy, delicious recipes that include casseroles, pastas, soups, stir-fries, and slow cooker meals. The book contains a collection of meals that are perfect for the cook who wants home-cooked, nutritious, fresh food fast. Each recipe is low in oxalates to help heal symptoms of bladder pain, kidney stones, irritable bowel syndrome, fibromyalgia, and pain associated with oxalate stone formation in other parts of the body. It's a prevention diet often recommended for kidney stone issues.

Index

Valentine's Day 2017

Dear Tim,

I look forward to making beautiful food with you, I hope you enjoy.

With Love,
 Eileen

Made in the USA
Lexington, KY
07 February 2017